# Physiology in Clinical Neurosciences – Brain and Spinal Cord Crosstalks

**Series Editor**
Hemanshu Prabhakar, Department of Neuroanesthesiology,
All India Institute of Medical Sciences, New Delhi, India

Central nervous system that includes brain and spinal cord has high metabolic demand. The physiology of the brain is such that it is easily affected by any altered physiology of other systems which in turn may compromise cerebral blood flow and oxygenation. Together the brain and spinal cord control our body systems to function automatically. While other systems of body controls individual functions, central nervous system at the same time does many different functions, especially, controlling the function of other systems. However, only little is known that central nervous system itself affects almost all the other systems of the body for example, cardiovascular, respiratory, renal, genitourinary, gastrointestinal, hematological etc. This interaction of brain and spinal cord with other systems makes it important for us to understand how any kind of injury to the central nervous system may at times, produce complications in remote organs or systems of the body. It is these lesser known crosstalks between acutely or chronically affected brain and spinal cord and other systems of the body that is discussed in this book series. Each system would be considered in a separate book.

Hemanshu Prabhakar • Manpreet Kaur
Editors

# Brain and Endocrine Crosstalk

Springer

*Editors*
Hemanshu Prabhakar
Department of Neuroanesthesiology and Neurocritical Care
All India Institute of Medical Sciences
New Delhi, Delhi, India

Manpreet Kaur
Department of Physiology
VMMC and Safdarjung Hospital
New Delhi, Delhi, India

ISSN 2524-8294 ISSN 2524-8308 (electronic)
Physiology in Clinical Neurosciences – Brain and Spinal Cord Crosstalks
ISBN 978-981-92-0762-6 ISBN 978-981-92-0763-3 (eBook)
https://doi.org/10.1007/978-981-92-0763-3



This Springer imprint is published by the registered company Springer Nature Singapore Pte Ltd.
The registered company address is: 152 Beach Road, #21-01/04 Gateway East, Singapore 189721, Singapore

*We dedicate this work to our teachers and mentors, whose wisdom, guidance, and encouragement have shaped our academic and professional journeys. Their passion for learning and commitment to excellence have inspired us to explore the fascinating interface between physiology, neuroscience, and endocrinology.*

*This book is also devoted to the students, scholars, and clinicians who dedicate themselves to advancing biomedical science and improving patient care. It is our hope that this work will support their curiosity, strengthen their understanding, and inspire further exploration in the rapidly evolving field of neuroendocrinology.*

*Above all, we dedicate this book to our parents and families, whose constant support, patience, and encouragement make every academic endeavor possible. Their belief in our work has been a source of strength and motivation throughout the process of bringing this book to completion.*

*With gratitude and respect, this book is offered to all who seek to deepen their understanding of the remarkable dialogue between the brain and the endocrine system, and to those committed to translating this knowledge into better health and well-being for humanity.*

*This book is for you.*

# Preface

The human body functions through an extraordinary network of regulatory systems that maintain internal balance and coordinate responses to internal and external stimuli. Among these, the endocrine and nervous systems form two of the most sophisticated and interconnected regulatory frameworks. Their dynamic interaction governs a wide spectrum of physiological processes, including metabolism, growth and development, reproduction, stress responses, and circadian rhythms. In recent decades, growing scientific understanding has revealed that these systems do not operate independently; rather, they engage in continuous and complex communication known as brain–endocrine cross-talk. This book has been developed to explore this fascinating interface, presenting a comprehensive account of the physiology and neurophysiology of the endocrine system and their clinical implications.

The objective of this book is to provide a structured and integrated understanding of neuroendocrinology, beginning with the foundational principles of endocrine physiology and progressing toward the intricate regulatory mechanisms linking the brain and endocrine organs. To facilitate this understanding, the book follows a three-tier approach. The first section introduces the core concepts of endocrine physiology, outlining the structure and function of endocrine glands and the mechanisms through which hormones regulate essential bodily functions. The second section focuses on the neurophysiology of the endocrine system, highlighting how neural pathways influence hormonal secretion and endocrine activity. The final section culminates in an in-depth exploration of the cross-talk between the brain and endocrine system, emphasizing how neural and hormonal signals integrate to maintain homeostasis and respond to physiological challenges.

The chapters of this book address several key topics central to contemporary neuroendocrinology. These include the physiological basis of endocrine function, endocrine control of metabolism, and modern diagnostic approaches to endocrine disorders. The text further examines the neural regulation of endocrine glands, the neuroendocrine response to stress, and the hormonal regulation of circadian rhythms. Special emphasis is placed on the complex bidirectional communication between neural and endocrine systems, illustrating how disruptions in these interactions contribute to a range of neuroendocrine disorders. In addition, the book highlights important clinical implications and discusses recent advances and emerging trends in neuroendocrine research.

This work is intended to serve as a valuable resource for a wide range of readers, including researchers, clinicians, postgraduate students, and super-specialty trainees in the fields of neuroscience, endocrinology, physiology, and biomedical sciences. By presenting fundamental principles alongside clinical perspectives, the book seeks to bridge the gap between basic science and medical practice. It aims to help readers understand the physiological basis of various neuroendocrine disorders and to support improved approaches to their diagnosis, assessment, and management.

Furthermore, the book emphasizes interdisciplinary learning by integrating concepts from physiology, neurology, endocrinology, and clinical medicine. Such integration is essential in today's rapidly advancing biomedical landscape, where collaborative knowledge drives innovation and improved patient care. By combining foundational science with contemporary research insights, the text encourages readers to explore the evolving dimensions of neuroendocrinology and appreciate its relevance in both academic and clinical contexts.

Ultimately, this book aspires to deepen understanding of the intricate dialogue between the brain and endocrine system. It aims to inspire curiosity, promote critical thinking, and equip readers with the knowledge necessary to explore novel therapeutic strategies and contribute meaningfully to the expanding field of neuroendocrinology.

New Delhi, Delhi, India Manpreet Kaur Ghai
New Delhi, Delhi, India Hemanshu Prabhakar

# Acknowledgments

We wish to acknowledge the support of the Administration of All India Institute of Medical Sciences (AIIMS), New Delhi (India), for allowing us to carry out this academic task.

We thank the faculty and staff in the Department of Neuroanaesthesiology and Neurocritical Care at AIIMS, New Delhi, for their support.

We would also like to acknowledge the support and encouragement received from the Administration and colleagues at the Department of Physiology, Vardhman Mahavir Medical College (VMMC) and Safdarjung Hospital, New Delhi.

Special thanks to the team of Springer for their assistance and guidance throughout the process.

Hemanshu Prabhakar
Manpreet Kaur

# Contents

**Part I Physiology of Endocrine Organs**

1 **An Introduction to Endocrine Physiology** ....................... 3
Kiran Prakash

2 **Hypothalamus and Pituitary** ....................... 11
Shival Srivastav

3 **Thyroid Gland** ....................... 25
Shival Srivastav

4 **Hormones in Calcium Homeostasis** ....................... 35
Manpreet Kaur and Kiran Prakash

5 **Adrenal Gland** ....................... 53
Manpreet Kaur

6 **Pineal Gland and Circadian Rhythms: Melatonin and Sleep–Wake Cycle Regulation** ....................... 79
Tania Talwar

7 **Endocrine Control of Metabolism: Hormonal Regulation of Energy Homeostasis** ....................... 101
Tania Talwar

8 **Diagnostic Approaches to Endocrine Disorders** ....................... 129
Kiran Prakash

**Part II Neurophysiology of Endocrine Organs**

9 **Introduction to Neuroendocrinology** ....................... 137
Kiran Prakash

10 **Neural Regulation of Endocrine System** ....................... 145
Mahesh Arjundan Gadhvi and Shival Srivastav

11 **Hypophysiotropic Neuroendocrine Axes and Neuroendocrine Regulation** ....................... 161
Bhawna Mattoo

**12 Neuroendocrine Adaptations to Physiological and Clinical Conditions** . . . 173
Manpreet Kaur

**Part III Brain and Endocrine Crosstalk**

**13 Brain and Endocrine Crosstalk: Clinical Implication for Neurocritical Care** . . . . . . . . . . . . . . . . . . . . . . . . . . . . . . . . . . . . . . . 189
Tulskii Ivan, Kulikov Alexander, and Savin Ivan

# Part I

# Physiology of Endocrine Organs

# An Introduction to Endocrine Physiology 1

Kiran Prakash


**Abstract**

The endocrine system regulates body functions via hormones from ductless glands. These glands include the hypothalamus, pituitary, thyroid, parathyroid, adrenals, pancreas, gonads, pineal gland, etc. These glands send signals over long distances by releasing secretions directly into the blood. These signals help control growth, metabolism, and homeostasis. The hypothalamus controls anterior pituitary tropic hormones (which affect the thyroid, adrenal glands, and gonads) and stores posterior hormones like oxytocin and vasopressin. The suprachiasmatic nucleus sets the body's circadian rhythms for cortisol and melatonin.

Hormones have strong, amplified effects at picomolar–nanomolar levels through specific receptors. The activation of receptors starts cascades or changes gene expression. Signaling can be endocrine (distant), paracrine (local), autocrine (self), or intracrine (inside the cell). Pulsatile release keeps sensitivity high, and receptor expression makes sure that tissues respond in different ways.

Peptides and proteins like thyrotropin-releasing hormone, insulin, and growth hormone use cell-surface receptors called G protein-coupled receptors and receptor tyrosine kinases. Adrenal and gonadal steroids like cortisol and testosterone bind to nuclear receptors to change genes. Catecholamines (epinephrine) come from amino acids through G protein-coupled receptors. Eicosanoids and vitamin D add paracrine and nuclear modes.



K. Prakash (✉)
Department of Physiology, Government Medical College and Hospital, Sector 32, Chandigarh, India







H. Prabhakar, M. Kaur (eds.), *Brain and Endocrine Crosstalk*, Physiology in Clinical Neurosciences – Brain and Spinal Cord Crosstalks,
https://doi.org/10.1007/978-981-92-0763-3_1

Negative feedback keeps levels steady. Positive loops regulate ovulation and parturition. Cells can directly control things like glucose and calcium by sensing them. Neural and immune integration makes this more accurate.

**Keywords**

Endocrine system · Hormones · Hypothalamic–pituitary axis · Negative feedback · Receptor signaling · Circadian rhythm · Homeostasis · Positive loops

## 1.1 Introduction

The endocrine system is the master system of controlling and regulating the body's functions. It allows hormones and chemicals to speak to each other over long distances through the blood in order to coordinate various body functions. The endocrine system works to keep the body balanced, by regulating growth, development, and metabolism [1, 2].

## 1.2 Endocrine System: Setup

Endocrine system is a network of specialized glands and hormone-producing tissues that are spread out across the body. The hypothalamus, pituitary gland (which has separate anterior and posterior lobes), thyroid and parathyroid glands, adrenal glands (cortex and medulla), pancreatic islets of Langerhans, gonads (ovaries and testes), and pineal gland are all examples of classical endocrine glands. These organs are called ductless glands because they release their secretions directly into the blood instead of through excretory ducts [1, 3].

Many tissues with other main jobs also are big players in controlling hormones. The heart releases atrial and brain natriuretic peptides. They regulate blood volumes and blood pressure [4]. Kidneys produce erythropoietin and also help to form the active form of vitamin D [5]. Adipose tissue generates hormones like leptin, adiponectin, and resistin [6]. The digestive system produces all kinds of other hormones—like gastrin, secretin, cholecystokinin, and ghrelin. They help to regulate digestion and keep the body's energy levels in balance [7].

## 1.3 Hierarchical Organization

One of the most important parts of the endocrine system is its ability to control things in a hierarchy. The hypothalamus is at the top. It puts together information about the brain, metabolism, and the environment. The hypothalamus controls the anterior pituitary gland's secretion by secretion of stimulatory and inhibitory hormones. After that, the anterior pituitary sends out tropic hormones. These tropic hormones make the thyroid, adrenal cortex, and gonads work harder [8, 9]. The posterior pituitary stores and releases oxytocin and vasopressin made in hypothalamic neurons. These neurons connect neural activity directly to the release of hormones throughout the body [10].

## 1.4 Integration of Functions

The endocrine system works closely with the nervous and immune systems to form a single regulatory network. Neural signals can directly cause hormone release, for example, sympathetic nervous system controls the release of catecholamines from the adrenal medulla [11]. The hypothalamus itself acts as a neuroendocrine interface, turning different neural signals into endocrine signals [8, 10]. The suprachiasmatic nucleus sends out circadian timing signals that make hormones, like melatonin from the pineal gland and daily changes in cortisol and other hormones, release in a rhythmic way [12].

## 1.5 Principles of Endocrine Function

Hormones are made and released in very small amounts, but they have strong and often long-lasting effects on the body. Hormones move through the bloodstream to reach faraway targets, while neurotransmitters work across tiny synaptic clefts. The cells with the compatible receptors interact with these neurotransmitters and respond specifically. Hormonal strength is very high. Effective concentrations are usually between picomolar and nanomolar, which shows that receptors have a high affinity for them and that there are strong intracellular amplification mechanisms. A single hormone molecule can start signaling cascades that make thousands of secondary messengers or change the transcription of many genes, greatly increasing the strength of the original signal [13, 14].

Classical endocrine signaling is when hormones travel through the blood to affect distant targets. Endocrine communication, on the other hand, includes many other ways of sending messages. Prostaglandins are an example of paracrine signaling, which affects cells that are close by in the same tissue. Intracrine signaling is when hormones act inside the cell that made them, without being released. Autocrine signaling is when cells control their own activity. Many hormones work in more than one way at the same time, which lets them coordinate at both the systemic and local levels [15].

This signaling versatility gives the endocrine system a lot of freedom. For example, insulin works throughout the body to control glucose metabolism and also has autocrine effects on pancreatic beta cells [16]. This kind of variety makes it possible for both global integration and precise local control.

## 1.6 Specificity Through Receptors

Receptor expression is what determines hormonal specificity. Hormones travel all over the body, but only cells that have the right receptor can respond to them. This rule explains why one hormone can cause different responses in different types of tissue. Testosterone increases muscle size, deepens the voice, and encourages hair growth by acting on the androgen receptor. The effects on different tissues depend on local cofactors and gene expression programs [17].

## 1.7 Time Dynamics

Hormonal signaling is always changing. Many hormones are released in a rhythmic or pulsing way that is necessary for normal function. Cortisol levels rise and fall with the circadian rhythm, reaching their highest point in the early morning [18]. During deep sleep, growth hormone is released in small bursts. In women, reproductive hormones change every month, and in both sexes, they pulse every few hours [19]. These time patterns make physiological responses work better and keep receptor sensitivity high.

## 1.8 Classification of Hormones: Based on Chemical Structures

Hormones are usually divided into groups based on their chemical nature. Each of which has a different site of synthesis and different receptors (Table 1.1).

Peptide and protein hormones make up the largest group. They include small peptides like thyrotropin-releasing hormone and large proteins like growth hormone and follicle-stimulating hormone. They are made as preprohormones, then processed in the endoplasmic reticulum and Golgi apparatus, stored in secretory vesicles, and released when needed. Because they dissolve in water, they can move around freely or be loosely bound. They have short half-lives and work through cell-surface receptors [20].

Cholesterol is the source of steroid hormones, which are made mostly in the adrenal cortex, gonads, and placenta. Their rate of secretion is determined by how quickly they are made, since they are not stored. Because they are lipophilic, they need carrier proteins to move around and can cross cell membranes and bind to intracellular receptors. This usually has genomic effects that last longer [21].

Hormones made from amino acids come from tyrosine or tryptophan. Peptide hormones act like catecholamines, and thyroid hormones act like steroids. Melatonin, which comes from tryptophan, is a key part of regulating circadian rhythms. This group shows that the chemical makeup does not always predict its mode of transport and action.

**Table 1.1** Chemical classification of hormones based on molecular structure

| Hormone class | Chemical nature | Representative examples | Primary site of synthesis | Receptor type |
|---|---|---|---|---|
| Peptide hormones | Short chains of amino acids | TRH, GnRH, vasopressin, oxytocin | Hypothalamus, pituitary, | Cell-surface (GPCRs) |
| Protein hormones | Long polypeptides | Insulin, growth hormone, prolactin | Pancreas, pituitary | Cell-surface (RTKs, JAK-STAT, GPCRs) |
| Glycoprotein hormones | Protein hormones with carbohydrate side chains | TSH, FSH, LH, hCG | Anterior pituitary, placenta | Cell-surface (GPCRs) |
| Steroid hormones | Cholesterol-derived lipophilic molecules | Cortisol, aldosterone, estradiol, testosterone, progesterone | Adrenal cortex, gonads, placenta | Intracellular nuclear receptors |
| Amino acid-derived (catecholamines) | Tyrosine derivatives | Epinephrine, norepinephrine, dopamine | Adrenal medulla, central nervous system | Cell-surface (GPCRs) |
| Amino acid-derived (iodothyronines) | Iodinated tyrosine residues | Thyroxine, triiodothyronine | Thyroid follicular cells | Intracellular nuclear receptors |
| Eicosanoids | Arachidonic acid metabolites | Prostaglandins, leukotrienes, thromboxanes | Most tissues | Cell-surface (GPCRs) |
| Vitamin-derived hormones | Modified vitamins | Calcitriol (vitamin D), retinoic acid | Skin, liver, kidney | Intracellular nuclear receptors |

*TRH* thyrotropin-releasing hormone, *GnRH* gonadotropin-releasing hormone, *GPCRs* G-protein coupled receptors, *RTKs* receptor tyrosine kinases, *JAK-STAT* Janus kinase's and signals transducer and activator of transcription proteins, *TSH* thyroid-stimulating hormone, *FSH* follicle-stimulating hormone, *LH* luteinizing hormone, *hCG* human chorionic gonadotropin

## 1.9 Classification Based on Function and Solubility

Hormones can also be grouped by their physiological role (e.g., metabolic regulators, growth and developmental hormones, reproductive hormones, stress-response hormones, water and electrolyte regulators, calcium, and bone regulators) (Table 1.2). Hormones that dissolve in water work through membrane receptors and second messengers. Hormones that dissolve in lipids mainly work through intracellular receptors and transcriptional regulation. These groups work together to help us understand how hormones work in healthy and unhealthy situations.

**Table 1.2** Classification of hormones based on functions and solubility

| Functional category | Physiological role | Representative hormones | Solubility |
|---|---|---|---|
| Metabolic regulators | Control energy balance, glucose, lipid, and protein metabolism | Insulin, glucagon, cortisol, thyroid hormones | Mixed (hydrophilic: insulin, glucagon; lipophilic: cortisol, T3, T4) |
| Growth and developmental hormones | Regulate somatic growth, tissue differentiation, maturation | Growth hormone, IGF-1, thyroid hormones | Hydrophilic (GH, IGF-1); lipophilic (T3/T4) |
| Reproductive hormones | Control gametogenesis, sexual differentiation, reproductive cycles | Estrogens, progesterone, testosterone, FSH, LH | Lipophilic (steroids); hydrophilic (FSH, LH) |
| Stress-response hormones | Mediate acute and chronic stress responses | Epinephrine, norepinephrine, cortisol | Hydrophilic (catecholamines); lipophilic (cortisol) |
| Water and electrolyte regulators | Maintain fluid balance, blood pressure, ion homeostasis | Aldosterone, vasopressin, ANP | Lipophilic (aldosterone); hydrophilic (vasopressin, ANP) |
| Calcium and bone regulators | Control calcium, phosphate, and bone remodeling | PTH, calcitriol, calcitonin | Hydrophilic (PTH, calcitonin); lipophilic (calcitriol) |

*IGF* insulin-like growth factor, *GH* growth hormone, *T3* triiodothyronine, *T4* thyroxine, *FSH* follicle-stimulating hormone, *LH* luteinizing hormone, *ANP* atrial natriuretic peptide, *ADH* antidiuretic hormone, *PTH* parathyroid hormone

## 1.10 Endocrine System Control: Negative Feedback

The main way to keep the endocrine system stable is through negative feedback. In these systems, the last hormone or its effect on the body stops the release of hormones higher up in the chain. This self-regulating design keeps hormone levels in a healthy range and can adapt to changing needs [22].

## 1.11 Endocrine System Control: Positive Feedback and Control of the Brain

Positive feedback loops are important for some biological events, even though they are rare. The estradiol-driven LH surge before ovulation [23] and the oxytocin-mediated contractions of the uterus during labor [24] are both examples of controlled positive feedback loops.

Neural regulation makes endocrine responses happen quickly. Direct sympathetic innervation of the adrenal medulla lets catecholamines be released under stressful conditions. Neurons in the hypothalamus make and release hormones from the posterior pituitary. The suprachiasmatic nucleus sends circadian signals that sync up endocrine rhythms with the light–dark cycle.

## 1.12 Hormonal Interactions and Substrate Sensing

Some endocrine cells can directly sense the components of blood, which lets them control things right away without needing other signals. Beta cells in the pancreas sense glucose [25], parathyroid cells sense calcium [7], and osmoreceptors in the hypothalamus control the release of vasopressin [10]. These self-contained feedback loops work with higher level regulatory systems. Pulsatile secretion fine-tunes the regulation. It maintains the receptor sensitivity. GnRH demonstrates that sustained exposure can paradoxically inhibit hormonal axes. This highlights the significance of temporal patterning [19].

## 1.13 Conclusion

The endocrine system is a good example of biological precision. It is set up in a hierarchy. Hormones use different methods to keep itself in check. Endocrine signaling coordinates physiology across different distances and time scales. For example, the hypothalamus–pituitary axes. To comprehend both normal physiology and endocrine disorders, it is essential to grasp the structure and operational principles of endocrine system.

The functional framework of the endocrine system serves as the foundation for research. Diabetes, thyroid disease, reproductive dysfunction, and metabolic syndrome exemplify disorders that exhibit issues with the principles delineated herein.

## References

1. Leblebicioglu B, Connors J, Mariotti A. Principles of endocrinology. Periodontol 2000. 2013;61(1):54–68.
2. Ukena K, Okada R. Recent advances in endocrine and neuroendocrine systems. Zoolog Sci. 2024;41(1):1–3.
3. Hiller-Sturmhöfel S, Bartke A. The endocrine system: an overview. Alcohol Health Res World. 1998;22(3):153–64.
4. Lugnier C, Meyer A, Charloux A, Andrès E, Gény B, Talha S. The endocrine function of the heart: physiology and involvements of natriuretic peptides and cyclic nucleotide phosphodiesterases in heart failure. J Clin Med. 2019;8(10):1746.
5. Acharya V, Olivero J. The kidney as an endocrine organ. Methodist Debakey Cardiovasc J. 2018;14(4):305–7.
6. Wozniak SE, Gee LL, Wachtel MS, Frezza EE. Adipose tissue: the new endocrine organ? A review article. Dig Dis Sci. 2009;54(9):1847–56.
7. Hong SH, Choi KM. Gut hormones and appetite regulation. Curr Opin Endocrinol Diabetes Obes. 2024;31(3):115–21.

8. Charlton H. Hypothalamic control of anterior pituitary function: a history. J Neuroendocrinol. 2008;20(6):641–6.
9. Hershman JM, Beck-Peccoz P. Discoveries around the hypothalamic-pituitary-thyroid axis. Thyroid. 2023;33(7):785–90.
10. Brown CH. Magnocellular neurons and posterior pituitary function. Compr Physiol. 2016;6(4):1701–41.
11. de Diego AMG, Gandía L, García AG. A physiological view of the central and peripheral mechanisms that regulate the release of catecholamines at the adrenal medulla. Acta Physiol (Oxf). 2008;192(2):287–301.
12. Chung S, Lee EJ, Cha HK, Kim J, Kim D, Son GH, et al. Cooperative roles of the suprachiasmatic nucleus central clock and the adrenal clock in controlling circadian glucocorticoid rhythm. Sci Rep. 2017;7:46404.
13. Evans RM, Mangelsdorf DJ. Nuclear receptors, RXR, and the big bang. Cell. 2014;157(1):255–66.
14. Lefkowitz RJ. Seven transmembrane receptors: something old, something new. Acta Physiol (Oxf). 2007;190(1):9–19.
15. Nussey S, Whitehead S. Principles of endocrinology. In: Endocrinology: an integrated approach [Internet]. BIOS Scientific Publishers; 2001 [cited 2025 Dec 30]. Available from: https://www.ncbi.nlm.nih.gov/books/NBK20/.
16. Petersen MC, Shulman GI. Mechanisms of insulin action and insulin resistance. Physiol Rev. 2018;98(4):2133–223.
17. Van-Duyne G, Blair IA, Sprenger C, Moiseenkova-Bell V, Plymate S, Penning TM. The androgen receptor. Vitam Horm. 2023;123:439–81.
18. Dickmeis T. Glucocorticoids and the circadian clock. J Endocrinol. 2009;200(1):3–22.
19. Stamatiades GA, Kaiser UB. Gonadotropin regulation by pulsatile GnRH: Signaling and gene expression. Mol Cell Endocrinol. 2018;463:131–41.
20. Hook V, Funkelstein L, Lu D, Bark S, Wegrzyn J, Hwang SR. Proteases for processing proneuropeptides into peptide neurotransmitters and hormones. Annu Rev Pharmacol Toxicol. 2008;48:393–423.
21. Miller WL, Auchus RJ. The molecular biology, biochemistry, and physiology of human steroidogenesis and its disorders. Endocr Rev. 2011;32(1):81–151.
22. Fekete C, Lechan RM. Central regulation of hypothalamic-pituitary-thyroid axis under physiological and pathophysiological conditions. Endocr Rev. 2014;35(2):159–94.
23. Herbison AE. Control of puberty onset and fertility by gonadotropin-releasing hormone neurons. Nat Rev Endocrinol. 2016;12(8):452–66.
24. Hamburg-Shields E, Mesiano S. The hormonal control of parturition. Physiol Rev. 2024;104(3):1121–45.
25. Henquin JC. Regulation of insulin secretion: a matter of phase control and amplitude modulation. Diabetologia. 2009;52(5):739–51.

# Hypothalamus and Pituitary

# 2

Shival Srivastav

**Abstract**

Crosstalk between the neural and endocrine systems plays an important role in the day-to-day homeostatic processes in human body. The endocrine 'orchestra' is dictated by an efficient conductor, the pituitary gland that releases multiple trophic hormones. These hormones act on target endocrine glands to release their respective hormones. The 'conductor' pituitary gland is efficiently managed by the hypothalamus, a part of diencephalon. The hypothalamus not only regulates the pituitary but also regulates multiple other body processes like appetite, thirst, temperature regulation and circadian rhythm. In the present chapter, we provide a brief overview of the hypothalamus and pituitary and discuss the physiological actions of these glands.

**Keywords**

Appetite regulation · Circadian rhythm · Endocrine system · Endocrine glands · Hypothalamus · Pituitary gland · Crosstalk · Trophic hormones

## 2.1 Hypothalamus

The hypothalamus is one of the key areas in forebrain having a pivotal role in homeostasis. By virtue of its vast connections with the periphery and its ability to receive diverse information via its afferents, hypothalamus is able to regulate diverse physiological functions of the human body. These functions consist of, but are not limited to, appetite and thirst, energy homeostasis, temperature regulation, sleep wake behaviour, sexual behaviour, response to stress and circadian rhythm. In addition, connections of hypothalamus with pituitary enable neuro-endocrine regulation

S. Srivastav (✉)
Department of Physiology, All India Institute of Medical Sciences, Jodhpur, Rajasthan, India
e-mail: srivastavs@aiimsjodhpur.edu.in



H. Prabhakar, M. Kaur (eds.), *Brain and Endocrine Crosstalk*, Physiology in Clinical Neurosciences – Brain and Spinal Cord Crosstalks,
https://doi.org/10.1007/978-981-92-0763-3_2

of physiological functions. The pivotal role of hypothalamus in these important physiological processes may be reason why it is one of the most conserved regions of the brain across multiple species when viewed from a phylogenetic perspective.

The word hypothalamus signifies its anatomical location, wherein "hypo" means below and "thalamus" denotes a key area of the brain. Wilhelm His is credited with devising the term 'hypothalamus' in the early 1890s [1]. Further work in this area was done by S. Ramon Y Cajal, and other scientists helped lay the foundation of the structural complexities and functional significance of this miniscule and seemingly trivial brain area.

## 2.2 Anatomy

The hypothalamus is a part of diencephalon of the brain. It forms a very small part of brain volume by mass (~0.5%) but has key roles to play in homeostasis. It is bound anteriorly by lamina terminalis and posteriorly by mamillary bodies. It lies below the thalamus, and a reasonable chunk of the organ surrounds the third ventricle.

The hypothalamus can be divided into four key areas along the rostro-caudal axis. These areas are chiasmatic (anterior), tuberal (middle) and mamillary (posterior). Each of these areas is divided into lateral, medial and periventricular zones [2]. Multiple nuclei are recognised in these areas that drive key physiological functions. A summary of the nuclei in different areas of hypothalamus is provided in Table 2.1.

## 2.3 Physiological Functions of Hypothalamus

### 2.3.1 Appetite and Feeding

The hypothalamus is the key area of the brain regulating appetite and feeding behaviour. The identification of this area as a key regulator of feeding behaviour dates back to the 1950s. Seminar experiments performed by Anand and colleagues [3–5] helped identify the importance of hypothalamus as a regulator of appetite. Electrolytic lesions were made in hypothalamus to study the effects on feeding.

**Table 2.1** Zones of hypothalamus and key nuclei

| Zone | Anterior | Middle | Posterior |
|---|---|---|---|
| Medial | Pre-optic | Dorsomedial | Posterior |
| | | Ventromedial | |
| | Suprachiasmatic | Arcuate | Mamillary |
| | Supra-optic | | |
| | Paraventricular | | |
| Lateral | Lateral | | |

The hypothalamus is divided into anterior, middle and posterior regions, each divided into medial and lateral zones. Key areas of these regions are shown in respective columns

Destruction of specific areas caused two mutually opposite behaviours—complete starvation and overeating. They observed that lesions in ventromedial area of hypothalamus (VMH) lead to a marked increase in appetite, whereas lesion in lateral hypothalamic area (LHA) was associated with cessation of feeding and food aversion. This was suggestive of the fact that VMH was a regulator of satiety, whereas LHA was associated with feeding behaviour. Therefore, a dual centre model was proposed based on these experiments. The interplay between feeding and satiety centres was said to govern feeding behaviour and thus determine the net energy intake. Earlier works proposed the mechanism of these areas working as an on/off switch, with the ability to start and stop feeding behaviour. However, the dual centre model was too simplistic to explain the different cues guiding feeding and satiety and complex feeding mechanisms.

With time, we came to realise that food intake may be governed by multitude of factors such as:

1. Blood glucose levels
2. Time of the day (circadian rhythms)
3. Gastrointestinal signals (governed by fed/fasting state)
4. Limbic system output, e.g. 'hedonic' or reward value of food
5. Energy stores in the body, e.g. body adipose tissue depot

Coexistence of multiple factors affecting feeding and satiety behaviour point to the intricate processing ability of the hypothalamic centres. To govern feeding and satiety behaviour, hypothalamus must be able to sense and process above-mentioned stimuli in real time. These signals may concomitantly emanate from different organ systems, thus pointing towards neurohumoral mechanisms relaying this information to the hypothalamus. Therefore the role of hypothalamus as a regulator of behaviour in response to food related cues is increasingly being recognised [6]. Hence its role extends well beyond the initiation and cessation of feeding. We have learnt that this area may have role in addiction and craving for sugar-rich foods [7].

Arcuate nucleus of hypothalamus (ARcH) plays a key role in regulation of feeding and metabolism. This area was initially named as 'nucleus infundibularis'. Two key classes of peptides—orexigenic and anorexigenic—are recognised. Arcuate nucleus receives signals from diverse regions of the brain.

### 2.3.2 Regulation of Thirst

Water constitutes approximately two-third of human body by weight. The osmolarities of different fluid compartments remain in close equilibrium and are tightly regulated so as to maintain homeostasis. Thirst is a fundamental homeostatic mechanism that helps the organism to maintain tonicity of body fluid compartments within normal range.

Multiple stimuli have been postulated for the sensation of thirst. Thirst may arise from oral signals such as mucosal dryness, visceral signals such as osmotic pressure

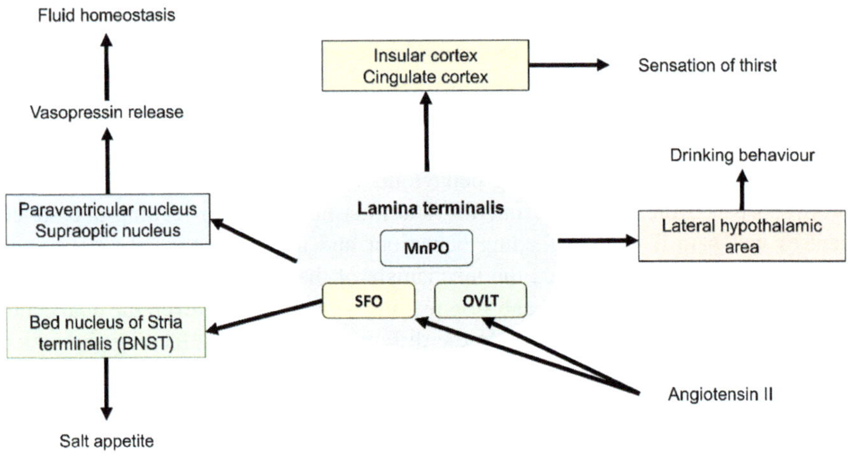


**Fig. 2.1** Central role of lamina terminalis in regulation of thirst. Lamina terminalis consists of median pre-optic area (MnPO), subfornical organ (SFO) and organum vasculosum of lamina terminalis (OVLT). While SFO and OVLT are outside blood–brain barrier and continuously sample ECF, they are well connected to MnPO. LT projects to different hypothalamic nuclei to regulate vasopressin release and fluid homeostasis, promote drinking behaviour and evoke sensation of thirst via insular and cingulate cortex. Angiotensin II also promotes thirst behaviour via signalling to SFO and OVLT. SFO also projects to BNST to promote salt seeking behaviour. (Figure based on information provided in Zimmerman [11], Rivera [10] and Wang [12])

in the GIT and circulating hormones such as angiotensin II [8]. Circumventricular organs, especially subfornical organ (SFO) and organum vasculosum of lamina terminalis (OVLT), have the ability to continuously sample body fluids so as to sense their tonicity. $Na_x$ channel in the circumventricular organs has been identified as the key player in the sensation of thirst [9]. SFO, OVLT and median pre-optic nucleus together form lamina terminalis, the central junction for regulation of fluid balance and homeostatic responses [10]. The connection of LT and its role in thirst regulation are summarised in Fig. 2.1.

### 2.3.3 Circadian Rhythm

Organisms on the Earth are entrained to 24-h day light cycle due to the length of the day. Circadian rhythms are biological cycles that occur on 24-h basis in healthy people. The word takes its origin from ‘circa diem’ which roughly translates to ‘about a day’. This periodicity in different physiological processes is critical to the survival. Circadian rhythms are based on “endogenous/internal” oscillators that are classified into central and peripheral oscillators. Suprachiasmatic nucleus (SCN) of the hypothalamus is the key central oscillator of the human body.

SCN receives day–night information from specialised cells in the retina. These cells are known as intrinsically photosensitive retinal ganglion cells (ipRGCs) [13].

A specialised tract, retino-hypothalamic tract, connects the retina to the SCN and conveys the day and night information to the SCN. The tract also synapses with multiple other areas of the hypothalamus. SNC expresses multiple clock genes that demonstrate rhythmic expression on a 24-h basis. These genes include CLOCK, BMAL, PER and CRY genes.

Two key transcription factors—circadian locomotor output cycles kaput (CLOCK) and brain and muscle aryl hydrocarbon receptor nuclear translocator-like protein 1 (BMAL1)—lead to the expression of PER and CRY genes. PER and CRY proteins formed as a result of this expression form a dimer and move to the nucleus and suppress their own transcription. Eventually, these proteins degrade after a 24 h period and restart the expression of CLOCK and BMAL1 genes, leading to rhythmicity associated with circadian rhythm [14, 15].

SCN also passes the circadian information to peripheral clocks by endocrine and systemic signals. Peripheral clock helps in synchronisation of different physiological processes like feeding, digestion, hormone secretion, fluid homeostasis and blood pressure perturbations in sync with the SCN [16, 17]. Thus, all the physiological processes of an organism are synchronised to 24-h cycle.

SCN also regulates the release of melatonin from the pineal gland. Tryptophan is the precursor for this molecule. Melatonin is responsible for a wide array of functions in the human body, ranging from detoxification to blood pressure regulation to promotion of sleep [18].

### 2.3.4 Temperature Regulation

Body temperature helps drive different metabolic and enzymatic processes in the body essential for maintenance of different physiological processes. It is divided into ‘core’ and ‘shell’ temperature which represent the temperature of internal viscera and superficial layers of the skin, respectively. While the shell temperature fluctuates according to the environment, core temperature is closely guarded and maintained in a very narrow range.

The pre-optic area (POA) of the hypothalamus is crucial to the maintenance of temperature. POA receives afferent information from core and shell regions of the body and generates compensatory responses to cold or warm temperatures. The sensation is perceived by thermoreceptors located in the periphery via transient receptor potential (TRP)-mediated signalling. The information is relayed by ascending pathways that enter via dorsal horn of the spinal cord. These signals traverse through the spinothalamic tract and reach the somatosensory cortex, providing the feeling of warmth or cold.

The signals also relay to the lateral parabrachial nucleus and reach the POA, which can initiate compensatory responses via descending spinal pathways. An overview of this information is provided in Fig. 2.2.

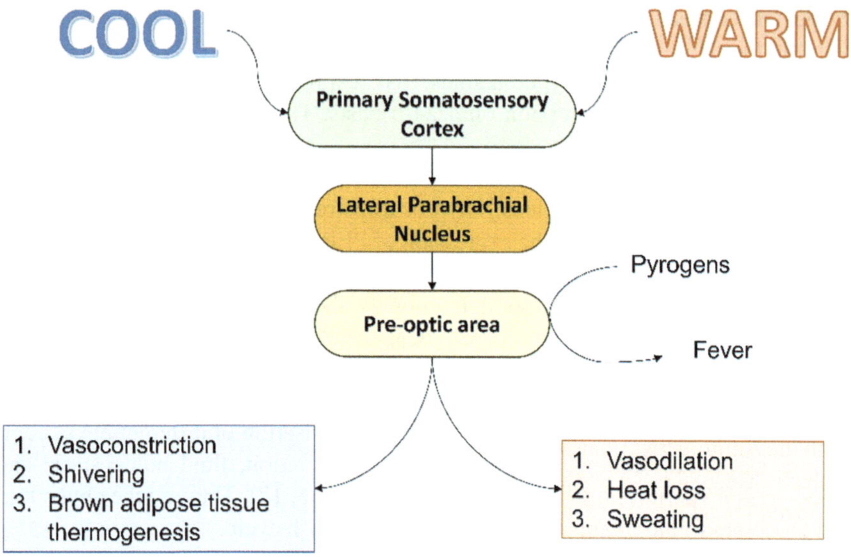


**Fig. 2.2** Thermoregulatory responses and the central role of pre-optic area (POA) [19–21]

**Table 2.2** Key hypophysiotropic hormones

| S. no | Hypophysiotropic hormones | Target cells in pituitary gland |
|---|---|---|
| 1 | Corticotropin releasing hormone | Corticotroph |
| 2 | Gonadotropin releasing hormone | Gonadotroph |
| 3 | Growth hormone releasing hormone | Somatotroph |
| 4 | Somatostatin | Somatotroph |
| 5 | Thyrotropin releasing hormone | Thyrotroph |

### 2.3.5 Regulation of Pituitary Function

Hypothalamus is the key regulator of the 'master of endocrine orchestra'—the pituitary gland. The pituitary gland consists of two parts—neurohypophysis and adenohypophysis. While the neurohypophysis is directly connected to the hypothalamus by means of descending projections, the adenohypophysis communicates with the hypothalamus by means of a portal system.

Hypothalamus releases a host of 'releasing' hormones that regulate the secretion of pituitary hormones. Important hypophysiotropic hormones are summarised in Table 2.2.

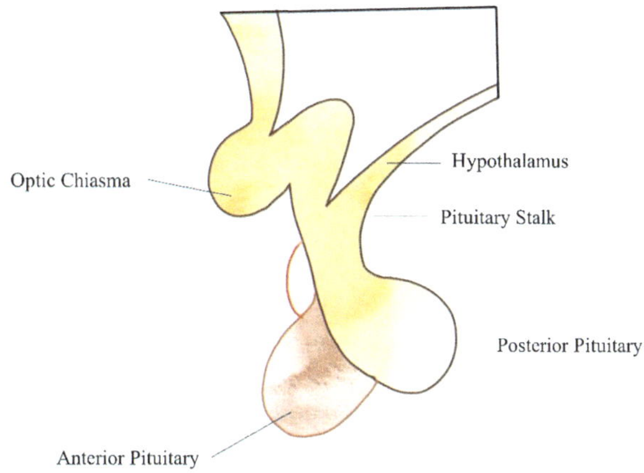


**Fig. 2.3** Schematic representation of pituitary gland

## 2.4 Pituitary Gland

Pituitary gland is the "master" endocrine gland in human physiology. Its importance can be understood by the fact that the hormones secreted by this gland are fundamental to the functioning of almost all major endocrine glands of human body. It is directly regulated by the hypothalamus, the 'controller of controllers'.

The word pituitary takes its roots from the Latin word 'pituita', meaning slime. There are two parts of this gland—anterior pituitary and posterior pituitary. The posterior pituitary is known as neurohypophysis, whereas the anterior part is known as neurohypophysis. Neurohypophysis is a direct extension of the diencephalon part of the brain, whereas adenohypophysis takes origin from 'Rathke's pouch', an outgrowth from oral ectoderm during the embryological period [22]. The gland is housed in 'sella turcica', a bony depression in the skull base. Figure 2.3 shows the anatomical structure of the pituitary gland.

The gland is stimulated by multiple releasing hormones released by the hypothalamus (Table 2.2) and in turn releases multiple 'trophic' hormones that act on multiple endocrine glands and stimulate them to release their hormones. These act in a negative feedback fashion with 'short' and 'long' feedback loops, thus establishing a delicate yet well-controlled feedback system to maintain the hormone levels within normal limits. This feedback hierarchy has been discussed by us previously [23, 24].

## 2.5 Key Hormones Released by Pituitary Gland and Their Actions

### 2.5.1 Growth Hormone

Growth hormone (GH) was discovered by Evans and Long [25], who demonstrated that extract from the anterior pituitary when administered intraperitoneally had a positive effect on the growth and oestrous cycle in rats. The hormone is produced by the 'somatotrophs' of the anterior pituitary gland. Its secretion is promoted by GHRH released from hypothalamus, while somatostatin inhibits the release of this hormone.

The GH receptor is a class I cytokine receptor and acts via JAK-STAT pathway. The earlier notion was GH binding caused dimerisation of two receptor subunits, leading of activation of signalling Janus family of kinases. However, this viewpoint has been challenged lately with the new view being that GH receptors exist as preformed dimers, with ach subunit being made up of an extracellular, a transmembrane and an intracellular domain [26, 27]. Activation of JAK2 causes phosphorylation of tyrosine residues and docking of STAT family of signalling proteins. Translocation of these STAT proteins to the nucleus leads to changes in gene expression and protein synthesis. Activation of MAP kinase pathway has also been proposed.

The actions of growth hormone are observed on multiple tissues. It acts on the skeleton to facilitate bone growth by acting on the growth plates located at the end of long bones. This action causes the proliferation and expansion of chondrocytes [28]. Also, an increase is observed in bone thickness and density.

On the metabolic front, GH has anti-insulin properties. It has a 'diabetogenic' effect leading to increase in blood glucose levels. It also regulates gluconeogenesis in the liver and causes conversion of white adipose tissue into brown adipose tissue and promotion of lipolysis.

GH also has positive immunological actions, wherein it promotes an increase in number of helper T cells. It is also shown to promote immune tolerance [29]. A number of actions of GH are mediated by insulin-like growth factors (IGFs), which act at tissue level and facilitate actions of GH.

GH deficiency leads to dwarfism and stunting of growth. Also observed are increased adipose tissue deposition and mental retardation. GH receptor deficiency can cause Levi Loran dwarfism. An excess of growth hormone leads to gigantism, if this happens before puberty. In adulthood, GH excess leads to acromegaly with thickening of bones and increase in bone density.

### 2.5.2 Prolactin

Prolactin (Prl) is synthesised in specialised cells of pituitary known as lactotrophs. The hormone is named so since it induced lactation after instillation of bovine extract in mammal research models. Like GH, the Prl receptor is also a member of class I cytokine superfamily with extracellular, transmembrane and intracellular segments [30]. Binding of the hormone to the receptor leads to phosphorylation of multiple intracellular proteins. STAT (signal transducer and activator of transcription) family proteins translocate to the nucleus to regulate gene expression.

Secretion of Prl hormone is negatively regulated by dopamine produced by the arcuate and paraventricular nucleus of hypothalamus. This is accomplished by downregulation of adenylate cyclase after dopamine binds to DR2 receptors on lactotrophes [31]. This reduced cAMP levels and interferes with nuclear signalling.

The primary action of Prl hormone is on the mammary gland, wherein this hormone induces gland development, milk formation and secretion. In animal models, Prl has been shown to maintain the structure and function of corpus luteum after mating. Also, it promotes nursing and nurturing behaviour by the mother for young pups. The effect on female sexual behaviour is controversial—while some studies report diminution, and others report increased sexual behaviour in female rats after instillation of this hormone in different brain areas.

In addition, Prl also shows other diverse actions such as immune regulation, osmoregulation and angiogenesis. The physiological effects of Prl and underlying mechanisms are well elaborated in Freeman et al. [32].

Physiological surges in levels of Prl are seen during breastfeeding, wherein stimulation of nipple by suckling leads to transient elevations. Stress and exercise can also lead to physiological elevations. However, pathological alterations may also be observed. Hyperprolactinemia can occur due to variety of reasons, with pituitary adenomas of lactotrophs and drug induced being the common causes. Antipsychotics are often associated with pathological elevations in Prl levels, and the treating physician should be vigilant towards this side effect. Long-term anti-epileptics and benzodiazepines may also cause this problem [31].

### 2.5.3 Follicle Stimulating Hormone (FSH) and Luteinising Hormone (LH)

FSH and LH are together known as gonadotropins since they are secreted by gonadotrophs of anterior pituitary. Both of them are heterodimeric glycoproteins in nature with two polypeptide units. These hormones share a common alpha subunit with thyroid stimulating hormone (TSH) and human chorionic gonadotropin (HCG), with beta subunits differing between the hormones [33]. This suggests that FSH and LH belong to a common family of hormones.

The release of FSH and LH is under hypothalamic control through a decapeptide hormone, gonadotropin releasing hormone (GnRH). The secretion of GnRH is pulsatile in nature, which helps regulate release of FSH and LH. Chronic infusion of this hormone leads to reduction in level of serum gonadotropins. Kisspeptin, a novel molecule, is responsible for this pulsatile release. The mechanism is shown in Fig. 2.4.

FSH, also known as follitropin, acts via G protein-coupled receptor FSHR. In females, FSH is primarily responsible for folliculogenesis in the ovary and synthesis of steroid hormones. FSH causes development of pre-antral follicles in the ovary eventually transforming them into antral follicles. Also, decreased expression of FSH receptors and reduced sensitivity to this hormone eventually result in atresia of non-dominant follicles and emergence of a dominant follicle which will undergo ovulation. FSH also increases the expression of LH receptors increasing the sensitivity of follicle to LH. In addition, FSH is said to play a role in ovulation process. These roles of FSH are well elaborated elsewhere [36–38]. The crosstalk between different types of ovarian cells and elaborate molecular mechanisms are discussed

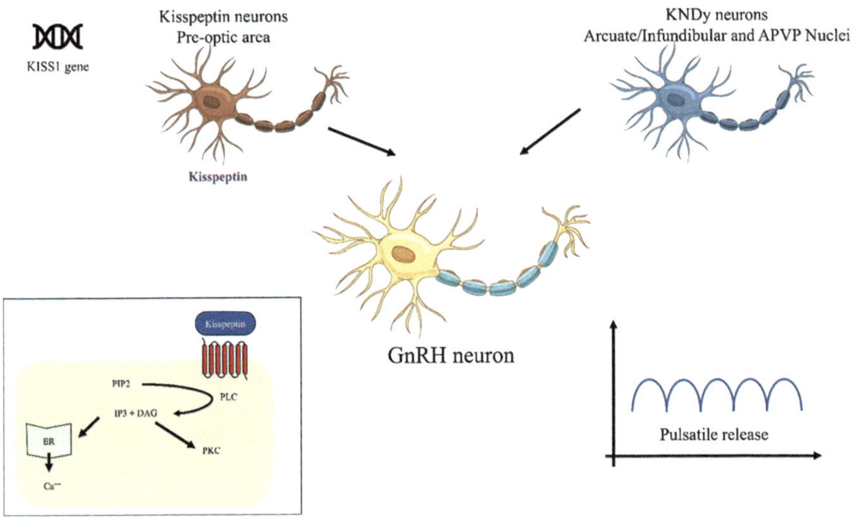


**Fig. 2.4** Kisspeptin and pulsatile release of GnRH [34, 35]. Kisspeptin is expressed in two key areas of hypothalamus—pre-optic area and arcuate nucleus (animals)/infundibular area (humans). KNDy neurons in arcuate nucleus co-express neurokinin and dynorphin. Together these two neuronal populations regulate GnRH release in pulsatile manner. Inset shows mechanism of action of kisspeptin through G protein-coupled receptor (GPCR), leading to dissociation of phospholipase C (PLC) into PIP2 and IP3 and DAG. DAG leads to activation of protein kinase C, whereas IP3 causes release of $Ca^{++}$ from endoplasmic reticulum and downstream actions. Image credits: NIAID Visual & Medical Arts (10/7/2024). Healthy neuron. NIAID NIH BIOART Source. bioart.niaid.nih.gov/bioart/197 and NIAID Visual & Medical Arts (5/13/2025). Receptor Protein. NIAID NIH BIOART Source. bioart.niaid.nih.gov/bioart/651

elsewhere [39]. In males, Sertoli cells express FSH receptors, and this hormone is known to control the maturation and division of Sertoli cells. Eventually, FSH also plays a role in spermatogenesis. In animal models, FSH has also been proposed to regulate bone health by its action on osteoclasts [40].

Luteinising hormone (LH) is responsible for the process of luteinisation, i.e. the conversion of ovarian follicles into 'corpus luteum', ready for ovulation. LH acts on two important cells—theca interna and granulosa cells in the ovary. LH acts on theca cells to promote the synthesis of male sex steroids, which then travel to the granulosa cells to be converted into oestradiol by the action of the enzyme aromatase. This production of oestrogen helps in the positive feedback cycle, which eventually leads to a massive increase in levels of LH hormone, known as 'LH surge'.

Another important role of LH is in the process of making the oocyte ready for fertilisation. The oocyte is trapped in the prophase I phase of cell cycle and cannot proceed with cell division. Under the influence of LH surge, the oocyte is able to proceed with meiosis I [36].

Together, FSH and LH are key hormones playing vital roles in reproductive physiology.

### 2.5.4 Oxytocin

Oxytocin is a nine amino acid long peptide (nonapeptide), which consists of a cyclic ring of 6 AA and a 3 AA tail. It was first synthesised and structure described by Vincent du Vigneaud. It differs from another hormone, vasopressin of posterior pituitary, by only 2 amino acids [41]. As discussed previously, these hormones are synthesised in magnocellular neurons of supra-optic and paraventricular nuclei of hypothalamus and are transported down into posterior pituitary for release.

It binds to its receptor, a seven transmembrane G protein-coupled receptor, leading to elevated intracellular $Ca^{++}$ levels via phospholipase C signalling. Oxytocin plays a major role in the process of child birth or 'parturition', wherein it promotes contraction of uterine myometrial cells, thereby assisting in delivery. In addition, it also promotes ripening of the cervix via prostaglandin-mediated mechanisms [42].

Another non-reproductive function of this hormone is in the neurobiology of motivation. The brain reward system resides in the meso-cortico-limbic system, which drives daily behaviours of reward and motivation. It has been shown that oxytocin increases the significance and the perception of stimuli that drive the motivational behaviour. It has been shown to promote bonding and drive sexual behaviour [43].

### 2.5.5 Vasopressin

Vasopressin is also known as arginine vasopressin or anti-diuretic hormone. It shares structural homology with oxytocin with difference in only two amino acids. Vasopressin binds to the V2 receptor located on collecting duct of human nephrons. Here it promotes the insertion of aquaporin molecules into the luminal epithelium, promoting the reabsorption of water and thereby producing concentrated urine (anti-diuretic effect) [44]. It also stimulates the reabsorption of sodium via epithelial sodium channels (ENaC) and regulates urea transport into interstitium. Together these factors also help fine-tune water reabsorption, the key function of this hormone.

In addition to renal actions, vasopressin also has diverse metabolic actions. It regulates urea synthesis in the liver and secretion of glucose regulating hormones from the pancreas and release of ACTH [45].

## 2.6 Summary

To summarise, together the hypothalamus and pituitary gland exert a delicate, yet efficient control over the endocrine system. This control system helps in efficient regulation of hormone secretion from different endocrine glands. In addition to its endocrine role, the hypothalamus also regulates multiple key processes such as feeding and drinking, temperature regulation and circadian rhythms.

## References


1. Kreier F, Swaab DF. History of hypothalamic research: 'The spring of primitive existence'. Handb Clin Neurol. 2021;179:7–43.
2. Fong H, Zheng J, Kurrasch D. The structural and functional complexity of the integrative hypothalamus. Science. 2023;382:388–94.
3. Anand BK, Brobeck JR. Localization of a 'feeding center' in the hypothalamus of the rat. Proc Soc Exp Biol Med Soc Exp Biol Med N Y N. 1951;77:323–4.
4. Anand BK, Chhina GS, Singh B. Effect of glucose on the activity of hypothalamic 'feeding centers'. Science. 1962;138:597–8.
5. Anand BK, Chhina GS, Sharma KN, Dua S, Singh B. Activity of single neurons in the hypothalamic feeding centers: effect of glucose. Am J Physiol. 1964;207:1146–54.
6. Sharpe MJ. The cognitive (lateral) hypothalamus. Trends Cogn Sci. 2024;28:18–29.
7. Qin D, Qi J, Shi F, Guo Z, Li H. About sugar addiction. Brain Behav. 2025;15:e70338.
8. Hiyama TY. Understanding of thirst in medical science. Yonago Acta Med. 2025;68:1–11.
9. Hiyama TY, Watanabe E, Ono K, Inenaga K, Tamkun MM, Yoshida S, et al. Nax channel involved in CNS sodium-level sensing. Nat Neurosci. 2002;5:511–2.
10. Encarnacion-Rivera L, Deisseroth K, Luo L. Neurobiology of thirst and hunger drives. Annu Rev Neurosci. 2025;48:381–403.
11. Zimmerman CA, Leib DE, Knight ZA. Neural circuits underlying thirst and fluid homeostasis. Nat Rev Neurosci. 2017;18:459–69.
12. Wang J, Lv F, Yin W, Gao Z, Liu H, Wang Z, et al. The organum vasculosum of the lamina terminalis and subfornical organ: regulation of thirst. Front Neurosci. 2023;17:1223836.
13. Bollinger T, Schibler U. Circadian rhythms—from genes to physiology and disease. Swiss Med Wkly. 2014;144:w13984.
14. Vitaterna MH, King DP, Chang AM, Kornhauser JM, Lowrey PL, McDonald JD, et al. Mutagenesis and mapping of a mouse gene, clock, essential for circadian behavior. Science. 1994;264:719–25.
15. Van Drunen R, Eckel-Mahan K. Circadian rhythms of the hypothalamus: from function to physiology. Clocks Sleep. 2021;3:189–226.
16. Dibner C, Schibler U, Albrecht U. The mammalian circadian timing system: organization and coordination of central and peripheral clocks. Annu Rev Physiol. 2010;72:517–49.
17. Pilorz V, Helfrich-Förster C, Oster H. The role of the circadian clock system in physiology. Pflugers Arch. 2018;470:227–39.
18. Reiter RJ, Tan DX, Galano A. Melatonin: exceeding expectations. Physiol Bethesda Md. 2014;29:325–33.
19. Morrison SF, Nakamura K, Madden CJ. Central control of thermogenesis in mammals. Exp Physiol. 2008;93:773–97.
20. Nakamura K. Central circuitries for body temperature regulation and fever. Am J Physiol Regul Integr Comp Physiol. 2011;301:R1207–28.
21. Nakamura K. Afferent pathways for autonomic and shivering thermoeffectors. Handb Clin Neurol. 2018;156:263–79.
22. Le Tissier PR, Hodson DJ, Lafont C, Fontanaud P, Schaeffer M, Mollard P. Anterior pituitary cell networks. Front Neuroendocrinol. 2012;33:252–66.
23. Prakash K, Kaur M, Srivastav S, Gadhvi M, Sharma R. 8—Neurophysiology of the endocrine system. In: Mahajan C, Kapoor I, Prabhakar H, editors. Brain and organ communication effects of crosstalk on neurophysiology. San Diego: Elsevier Inc.;2025. pp. 139–53.
24. Kaur M, Prakash K, Srivastav S, Gadhvi M, Sharma R. 9—Crosstalk between brain and the endocrine system. In: Mahajan C, Kapoor I, Prabhakar H, editors. Brain and organ communication effects of crosstalk on neurophysiology. San Diego: Elsevier Inc.; 2025. pp. 155–76.
25. Evans HM, Long LA. The effect of the anterior lobe of the hypophysis administered intraperitoneally upon growth and maturity and estrous cycles of the rat. Anat Rec. 1921;21:62.

26. Waters MJ, Brooks AJ. JAK2 activation by growth hormone and other cytokines. Biochem J. 2015;466:1–11.
27. Waters MJ. The growth hormone receptor. Growth Horm IGF Res Off J Growth Horm Res Soc Int IGF Res Soc. 2016;28:6–10.
28. Dixit M, Poudel SB, Yakar S. Effects of GH/IGF axis on bone and cartilage. Mol Cell Endocrinol. 2021;519:111052.
29. Frago LM, Chowen JA. Basic physiology of the growth hormone/insulin-like growth factor axis. Adv Exp Med Biol. 2005;567:1–25.
30. Harris J, Stanford PM, Oakes SR, Ormandy CJ. Prolactin and the prolactin receptor: new targets of an old hormone. Ann Med. 2004;36:414–25.
31. Haidenberg-David F, Sidauy-Adissi J, Moscona-Nissan A, Jonguitud-Zumaya E, Fugarolas-Morinelli M, Martinez-Mendoza F, et al. Overview of hyperprolactinemia: general approach and reproductive health implications. Arch Med Res. 2024;55:103102.
32. Freeman ME, Kanyicska B, Lerant A, Nagy G. Prolactin: structure, function, and regulation of secretion. Physiol Rev. 2000;80:1523–631.
33. Lizneva D, Rahimova A, Kim S-M, Atabiekov I, Javaid S, Alamoush B, et al. FSH beyond fertility. Front Endocrinol. 2019;10:136.
34. Koysombat K, Tsoutsouki J, Patel AH, Comninos AN, Dhillo WS, Abbara A. Kisspeptin and neurokinin B: roles in reproductive health. Physiol Rev. 2025;105:707–64.
35. Xie Q, Kang Y, Zhang C, Xie Y, Wang C, Liu J, et al. The role of kisspeptin in the control of the hypothalamic-pituitary-gonadal axis and reproduction. Front Endocrinol. 2022;13:925206.
36. Thomas C. Ovulation: a cellular symphony in three movements. Semin Cell Dev Biol. 2025;174:103634.
37. de Medeiros SF, Barbosa BB, de Medeiros MAS, Yamamoto MMW. Morphology and biochemistry of ovulation. Rev Bras Ginecol E Obstet Rev Fed Bras Soc Ginecol E Obstet. 2021;43:480–6.
38. Richards JS, Pangas SA. The ovary: basic biology and clinical implications. J Clin Invest. 2010;120:963–72.
39. Orozco-Galindo BV, Sánchez-Ramírez B, González-Trevizo CL, Castro-Valenzuela B, Varela-Rodríguez L, Burrola-Barraza ME. Folliculogenesis: a cellular crosstalk mechanism. Curr Issues Mol Biol. 2025;47:113.
40. Das N, Kumar TR. Molecular regulation of follicle-stimulating hormone synthesis, secretion and action. J Mol Endocrinol. 2018;60:R131–55.
41. Uvnäs-Moberg K. The physiology and pharmacology of oxytocin in labor and in the peripartum period. Am J Obstet Gynecol. 2024;230:S740–58.
42. Camerino C. The new frontier in oxytocin physiology: the oxytonic contraction. Int J Mol Sci. 2020;21:5144.
43. Love TM. Oxytocin, motivation and the role of dopamine. Pharmacol Biochem Behav. 2014;119:49–60.
44. den Ouden DT, Meinders AE. Vasopressin: physiology and clinical use in patients with vasodilatory shock: a review. Neth J Med. 2005;63:4–13.
45. Bankir L, Bichet DG, Morgenthaler NG. Vasopressin: physiology, assessment and osmosensation. J Intern Med. 2017;282:284–97.

# Thyroid Gland

# 3

Shival Srivastav

**Abstract**

The thyroid gland, taking its name from 'thyreos', is a shield-shaped gland located in front and below the larynx. The gland is made up of follicles filled up with colloid. These follicles synthesise thyroid hormones—tri-iodothyronine and tetra-iodothyronine, which control key metabolic functions in the human body. In addition, they also control neural and cardiovascular functions and play strong roles in neurodevelopment as well. Thyroid gland pathologies present commonly to the clinics and are important from a burden of disease perspective. In the present chapter, we provide an overview of the gland, structure–function relationship, key actions of its hormones and common pathologies presenting to the clinics.

**Keywords**

Endocrine physiology · Thyroid hormone receptors · Thyroid gland · Thyroid hormones · Tri-iodothyronine · Tetra-iodothyronine · Biosynthesis · Metabolism · Physiological actions

## 3.1 Anatomy: Structure–Function Relationship

The thyroid gland is located in the anterior part of the neck in antero-inferior relation to the larynx. The gland is enclosed in fascia. It derives its' arterial blood supply from superior and inferior thyroid arteries. These arteries arise from external carotid and subclavian artery, respectively. The venous drainage occurs by means of superior, middle and inferior thyroid vein, which eventually drains into the external jugular vein. The gland has a high vascularity that facilitates the synthesis and release of thyroid

S. Srivastav (✉)
Department of Physiology, All India Institute of Medical Sciences, Jodhpur, Rajasthan, India
e-mail: srivastavs@aiimsjodhpur.edu.in


H. Prabhakar, M. Kaur (eds.), *Brain and Endocrine Crosstalk*, Physiology in Clinical Neurosciences – Brain and Spinal Cord Crosstalks,
https://doi.org/10.1007/978-981-92-0763-3_3

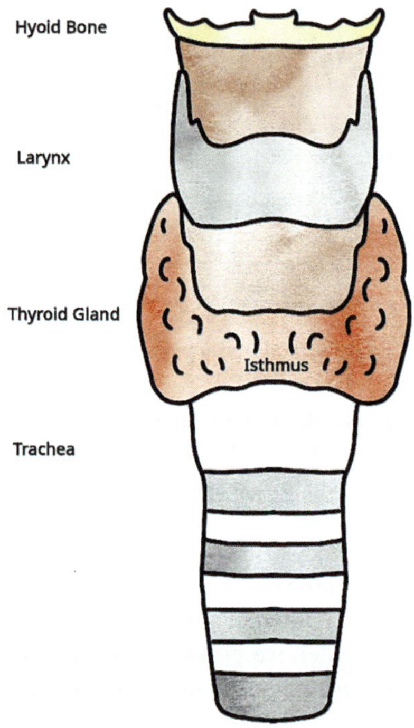


**Fig. 3.1** Anatomy of thyroid gland. The thyroid gland consists of two lobes, right and left connected together by an isthmus. The branches of external carotid and subclavian artery provide arterial supply (not shown), responsible for high vascularity of thyroid gland

hormones into the circulation. Thyroid gland consists of two lobes that are connected to each other via an isthmus. Gross anatomy of thyroid gland is shown in Fig. 3.1.

From a histological perspective, the gland is divided into multiple follicles. The follicles consist of a proteinaceous material filling its cavities, known as 'colloid'. The follicular epithelium is flattened in appearance in inactive follicles, whereas it assumes a columnar/cuboidal histology in active follicles. The colloid consists of thyroglobulin (Tg) protein, which acts as a binding protein for the purpose of storage of thyroid hormones. The relevance of thyroglobulin molecule shall be discussed shortly.

## 3.2 Thyroid Hormones: Synthesis

The thyroid gland releases two hormones, T3 (tri-iodothyronine) and T4 (tetra-iodothyronine or thyroxine). The hormones T3 and T4 are formed by the iodination of the tyrosine residues of thyroglobulin (Tg) protein. The synthetic process is summarised in Fig. 3.2.

The synthesis of thyroid hormones takes place in the follicular cells of the thyroid gland. Transport of iodine occurs via sodium-iodine symporter (Na-I Sym) located on the basal aspect of the cell. Since sodium is accumulated in the cell as a result of symport, there needs to exist a mechanism to extrude sodium out of cell and maintain the gradient for sodium inflow. This is accomplished by Na-K ATPase

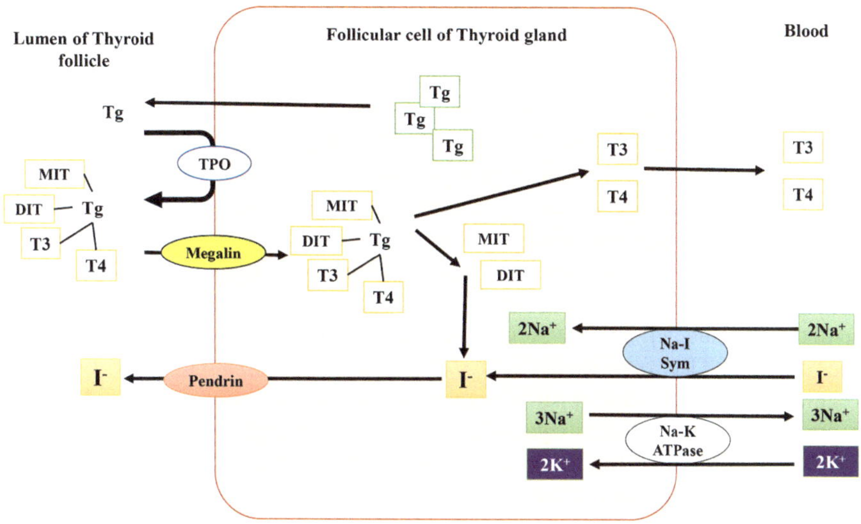


**Fig. 3.2** Biosynthesis of thyroid hormones in follicular cell. The diagram shows key steps in the biosynthesis of thyroid hormones in the follicular cell of thyroid gland. *Tg* thyroglobulin, *TPO* thyroid peroxidase, *MIT* monoiodotyrosine, *DIT* diiodotyrosine, *Na-I Sym* sodium-iodine symporter, *T3* triiodothyronine, *T4* tetraiodothyronine

pump, which pumps three sodium ions in lieu of two potassium ions. This electrogenic nature of Na-K ATPase maintains a negative balance for sodium ions inside the cell and therefore facilitates the operation of Na-I Sym. Once iodine ions enter the cell, they are extruded to the luminal compartment via a protein pump known as 'Pendrin'. The iodine, thus extruded, binds to tyrosine residues on the Tg protein—a process known as organification. This process is facilitated by thyroid peroxidase (TPO) enzyme. Addition of iodine to the tyrosine residues leads to the formation of monoiodotyrosine (MIT) or diiodotyrosine (DIT), depending on the number of additions. Post-formation of MIT and DIT, another reaction termed as 'coupling' takes place. Coupling of two DIT molecules leads to formation of T4 (tetra-iodothyronine), whereas coupling of MIT and DIT molecules leads to formation of T3 (tri-iodothyronine). The 'coupling' reaction is also catalysed by TPO enzyme.

Post-formation of hormones on the Tg molecule, the complex enters the thyroid cell through 'Megalin' transporter. Inside the follicular cell, the TG complex is broken down by lysosomal enzymes to release all above-mentioned iodinated products. T3 and T4 are released into the circulation, whereas MIT and DIT are acted upon by deiodinases, and the iodine thus released is sent for recycling.

## 3.3 Control of Thyroid Hormone Release

The release of thyroid hormones is controlled by the thyroid-stimulating hormone (TSH), which is released from the anterior pituitary gland. TSH is, in turn, under the influence of thyroid-releasing hormone (TRH). TRH is released from the cells of the paraventricular nucleus (PVN) of the hypothalamus. TRH is a tripeptide formed by the post translational processing of a 'prepro' hormone (13). The release of TRH from the PVN is under the influence of other higher centres of the brain. As we will discuss ahead, the thyroid hormones have a key role in regulation of different metabolic pathways and regulation of basal metabolic rate (BMR) in the body. Therefore, hypothalamic nuclei, namely arcuate nucleus and dorso-medial nucleus, influence the release of TRH from the PVN (13). These nuclei have an important role in the regulation of satiety and appetite regulatory mechanisms. In addition, adrenergic inputs from the medulla oblongata also influence TRH secretion—probably serving to regulate BMR and thermogenesis in the body. A detailed description of these influences and underlying mechanisms can be found elsewhere [1].

## 3.4 Protein Binding of Thyroid Hormones

Thyroid hormones are bound to three key proteins: thyroid-binding globulin (TBG), transthyretin and albumin.

## 3.5 Metabolism of Thyroid Hormones

T3 is the active form of thyroid hormone that binds to the thyroid receptor. But the predominant form of thyroid hormone in the circulation is T4. Therefore, for the purpose of hormone action at receptor level, one molecule of iodine needs to be removed from T4. This is accomplished by peripheral enzymes known as deiodinases. The iodine molecule can be removed from outer or inner ring. While the deiodination of outer ring T4 forms T3, inner ring deiodination forms reverse T3 (rT3), an inactive metabolite [2]. Three deiodinase forms are described, which act at different tissues to metabolise thyroid hormones. Type 1 and 2 deiodinases (D1 and D2) cause the conversion of T4 to T3, whereas Type 3 deiodinase (D3) causes the inactivation of thyroid hormones.

Other important pathways of thyroid hormone metabolism are sulphation, glucuronidation and deamination [2].

## 3.6 Thyroid Hormone Receptors

Two thyroid hormone receptor (THR) proteins have been described in literature: THR-$\alpha$ and THR-$\beta$. These proteins are coded by two distinct genes, THRA and THRB, respectively. These THRs are part of a larger nuclear receptor family, which

**Table 3.1** Thyroid receptor isoforms and expression[a]

| S. no. | Thyroid receptor isoform | Expression |
|---|---|---|
| 1. | Thyroid receptor-α1 and α2 | Brain (highest expression)<br>Kidney, skeletal muscle, heart, lungs, liver |
| 2. | Thyroid receptor-β1 | Kidneys, liver, heart, thyroid |
| 3. | Thyroid receptor-β2 | Brain, retina, inner ears |

[a]Information summarised from Refs. [4–9]

also includes oestrogen receptor and vitamin D receptor [3, 4]. Different isoforms of thyroid receptors exist. Their subtypes and locations are summarised in Table 3.1.

The hormone receptor consists of three functional domains [10]:

1. Amino terminal domain (A-B domain)
2. DNA binding domain (DBD)
3. Carboxyl-terminal ligand-binding domain (LBD)

Binding of the T3 hormone to the receptor leads to a change in the confirmation of the receptor, allowing it to bind to co-activator or co-repressor molecules [10]. Once the T3-hormone receptor complex is formed, it translocates to the nucleus to bind to the hormone response element of the nuclear DNA. This results in enhanced protein translation leading formation of proteins that act as effectors of thyroid hormone action. It is noteworthy that binding of co-activator molecules, such as p300 and steroid receptor co-activator-1 (SRC-1), is responsible for the increased avidity of binding [11, 12]. Conversely, co-repressor molecules may act to reduce protein transcription by decreasing the activity.

Recently, non-genomic mechanisms of thyroid hormone actions have also been discovered. Plasma membrane integrin receptor (αvβ3) serves as a cell surface receptor for thyroid hormones. T3 and T4 have been demonstrated to act via this receptor to promote angiogenesis and multiplication of tumour cells [13]. In addition to this integrin molecule, additional receptors may also be localised in the cytoplasm or on the plasma membrane, playing an important role in the non-genomic effects of the thyroid receptors. Downstream signalling pathways include MAP-kinase and Akt [11]. Previously, T4 was considered to be an intermediary that eventually got converted to T3 to exert its actions. The discovery of non-genomic pathways of thyroid hormone action, especially via MAP Kinase pathway, has brought forward the importance of T4 as an active hormone [14].

## 3.7 Physiological Actions of Thyroid Hormones

### 3.7.1 Action on the Nervous System

It is a well-established fact that thyroid hormones have a fundamental role in neural development. Congenital hypothyroidism is an important cause of mental retardation observed in patients with cretinism.

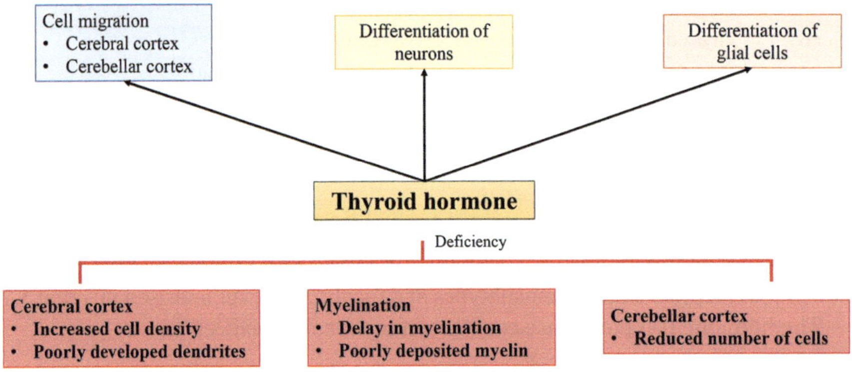


**Fig. 3.3** Summary of effects of thyroid hormone on neural development. (Adapted from information available in Bernal (2005), Berbel et al. (2001) and Pascual et al. (2013) [14–16])

Thyroid hormones have an important role for the division of neuronal cells and their myelination during early stage of life. Deficiency of thyroid hormones during the critical period of early brain development may lead to disruption of tissue organisation and architecture, with a potential adverse impact on overall neural function. A summary of effects of thyroid hormones on brain development is presented in Fig. 3.3. It is noteworthy that information is primarily sourced from experiments done on animal models, especially rat [14].

Deficiency of thyroid hormone leads to impaired neurogenesis, especially in the young age. While foetal thyroid function becomes functional at around 16–20 weeks of gestational age, physiological effects of thyroid hormones on neurogenesis are evident even before this period [17]. The source of thyroid hormones before the maturation of foetal thyroid function is from maternal circulation. Reduction in the levels of thyroid hormones during the critical window of neurogenesis has profound effects of neuronal division, migration and connectivity. Myelination of neurons is also impaired due to interference with oligodendrocyte function. In addition, interneurons in key brain areas may be affected, leading to poor neuronal connectivity, thus impairing overall brain function [17].

In adults, thyroid hormones are responsible for promotion of alertness and wakefulness. Increased memory and learning capacity with maintenance of normal emotional affect is also sub-served by thyroid hormones. In the peripheral nervous system, increased speed and amplitude of reflexes is observed.

### 3.7.2 Actions on Metabolic Pathways

As discussed previously, the balance between energy intake and expenditure governs the net energy depots and weight of an individual. The net energy expenditure depends on the sum of basal metabolic rate (BMR), physical activity and specific dynamic action of food. Thyroid hormones are important determinants of basal metabolic rate, as increased levels of thyroid hormones can lead to increased breakdown of cellular substrates to produce energy.

Thyroid hormones promote non-shivering thermogenesis by promoting the expression on uncoupling protein (UCP) in the mitochondria leading to dissociation of mitochondrial oxidative reactions and ATP formation. Therefore, the net reaction culminates in the production of heat energy without synthesis of ATP. This process takes place due to increased expression of UCP1 in the brown adipose tissue (BAT), promoted by T3 hormone. Also, thyroid hormones promote the conversion of white adipose tissue (WAT) into BAT, a process known as 'browning' of adipose tissue. Both the chemical processes—non-shivering thermogenesis and 'browning'—are promoted by increased sympathetic nervous system (SNS) activation [18].

Thyroid hormone also acts centrally at different hypothalamic nuclei leading to multiple physiological effects. An increased in body temperature is observed in addition to enhanced sympathetic outflow to BAT. Also, thyroid hormones are shown to promote feeding behaviour, probably due to increased expression of orexigenic peptides in the hypothalamic areas associated with feeding and satiety behaviour [18].

Thyroid hormones promote the turnover of glucose and also its catabolism for the purpose of energy generation. In the adipose tissue, thyroid hormones promote lipolysis and increase the mobilisation of free fatty acids (FFAs) from adipose tissue depots and dietary sources. These FFAs are taken up by the liver through increased expression of protein transporters in the liver. In addition, mobilisation of carbohydrates may also take place, diverting them towards synthesis of FFAs. These FFAs are eventually converted to triacylglycerols (TAGs) in the body [19].

### 3.7.3 Action on Musculoskeletal System

The thyroid hormones have an important role in maintenance of musculoskeletal health. Thyroid hormones (T3 and T4) have predominant actions on osteoblasts. The transport of thyroid hormones to the cells takes place via multiple transporters such as organic anion transporter protein 1c1 and monocarboxylate transporter 8 and 10 [20]. The effect of thyroid hormones on bone health varies with age. They promote bone growth and mineral deposition in young individuals, whereas, in the adult skeleton, thyroid hormones promote osteoclastic activity, thus enhancing bone resorption [20]. Increased thyroid hormone levels are associated with osteoporosis and increased probability of fractures [21].

Similarly, skeletal muscle is another important target of thyroid hormones. Thyroid hormones promote the division and differentiation of myoblasts during the initial phase of life. In addition, increased muscle contractility and relaxation are observed. Heat production by catabolism of energy substrates is promoted by thyroid hormones [16].

### 3.7.4 Action on Cardiovascular System

Thyroid hormones are responsible for maintenance of cardiovascular function. They have positive ionotropic and chronotropic effects, leading to increased rate and force of contraction. Right from the foetal life, thyroid hormones are responsible for promoting maturation of cardiac function. This occurs via increased transcription of genes encoding for adult variant of myocardial proteins, especially myosin-heavy chain [16]. Also, thyroid hormones are shown to enhance the expression of key molecules/receptors in the myocardium, such as Na-K ATPase, SERCA-2 and β1-adrenergic receptors. Thus, there is a positive effect on cardiac function.

A comprehensive list of thyroid hormone receptors, TR-α and -β, responsible for growth and differentiation of various cell types can be found in the literature [16].

## 3.8 Disorders of Thyroid Hormones

Disorders of thyroid hormones may be classified into two major categories—hyperthyroidism and hypothyroidism. Both entities may be subclinical or may present with frank clinical symptoms. Common causes of hyper- and hypo-thyroidism are summarised in Table 3.2.

Hyperthyroidism is characterised by classical clinical features of weight loss, diaphoresis, intolerance to hot temperature, anxiety and irritability. Increased futile cycles caused by the hormone are responsible for the high metabolic rate leading to many of the clinical features of the disorder. Grave's disease is amongst the commonest cause of hyperthyroidism seen in the elderly population. The disease is characterised by presence of thyroid stimulating antibodies (IgG) that provide continued stimulation of the gland leading to increased secretion of thyroid hormones into the circulation. The disease may also present with characteristic features of ophthalmopathy and dermopathy. Grave's ophthalmopathy is characterised by protrusion of eyeballs (exophthalmos), swelling of extra-ocular muscles and orbital contents, lid lag and retraction and congestion of conjunctiva. Due to persistent exposure of the corneal surface, drying of eyes followed by keratitis may be observed. In the long run, visual acuity may suffer if the condition is left untreated. Grave's dermopathy is seen around the shin, wherein the skin appears thickened and

**Table 3.2** Common causes of hyperthyroidism and hypothyroidism

| Hyperthyroidism | Hypothyroidism |
|---|---|
| 1. Grave's disease | 1. Hashimoto's disease |
| 2. Congenital | 2. Radioactive iodine therapy |
| 3. Toxic goitre | 3. Post-surgical |
| 4. Subacute thyroiditis | 4. Drug induced |
| 5. Drug induced | 5. Iodine deficiency |
| | 6. Neonatal |

Adapted from information provided in Refs. [21, 22]

like an orange peel. This occurs due to deposition of glycosaminoglycans in the pretibial region, hence the name pretibial myxoedema.

Another important cause of hyperthyroidism is thyroid adenoma, which may be single or present in clusters. Toxic goitre can result from single adenoma or multinodular goitre, wherein these nodules behave as autonomous entities secreting thyroid hormones into the circulation.

Subacute thyroiditis (also known as deQuervain's thyroiditis) occurs due to inflammation of the thyroid gland, often secondary to viral infections. The gland becomes swollen and painful, releasing copious amounts of thyroid hormones into the circulation. Post-inflammatory phase may present with reduced glandular function, leading to transient hypothyroidism.

Hypothyroidism is characterised by clinical features of weight gain, lethargy, intolerance to cold temperature, constipation, poor appetite and hoarseness of voice. Hashimoto's disease is one of the leading causes of hypothyroidism, wherein autoimmune destruction of the gland takes place. The gland is attacked by mononuclear immune cells, especially lymphocytes, leading to follicular infiltration and destruction [22]. Antibodies to thyroid antigens (especially thyroperoxidase and thyroglobulin) can be observed in circulation. Any insult to the gland, surgical or pharmacological, may also result in hypothyroidism. Administration of radioactive iodine, antithyroid drugs or neck irradiation may lead to reduction in glandular volume and function. Such intervention may also lead to hypothyroidism.

## 3.9 Summary

The thyroid gland synthesises T3 and T4 hormones that regulate key metabolic processes in the body. These hormones are vital to neurodevelopmental outcomes early in life and deficiency manifests in form of cretinism. In adults, alterations in these hormones may be seen due to a variety of pathologies and constitute an important disease burden. Thankfully, thyroid diseases are easily treatable given the rapid strides made in diagnosis and management of these disorders.

## References

1. Chiamolera MI, Wondisford FE. Minireview: thyrotropin-releasing hormone and the thyroid hormone feedback mechanism. Endocrinology. 2009;150:1091–6.
2. Van Drunen R, Eckel-Mahan K. Circadian rhythms of the hypothalamus: from function to physiology. Clocks Sleep. 2021;3:189–226.
3. Ortiga-Carvalho TM, Sidhaye AR, Wondisford FE. Thyroid hormone receptors and resistance to thyroid hormone disorders. Nat Rev Endocrinol. 2014;10:582–91.
4. Cheng S-Y, Leonard JL, Davis PJ. Molecular aspects of thyroid hormone actions. Endocr Rev. 2010;31:139–70.
5. Jones I, Ng L, Liu H, Forrest D. An intron control region differentially regulates expression of thyroid hormone receptor beta2 in the cochlea, pituitary, and cone photoreceptors. Mol Endocrinol Baltim Md. 2007;21:1108–19.

6. Ying H, Suzuki H, Zhao L, Willingham MC, Meltzer P, Cheng S-Y. Mutant thyroid hormone receptor beta represses the expression and transcriptional activity of peroxisome proliferator-activated receptor gamma during thyroid carcinogenesis. Cancer Res. 2003;63:5274–80.
7. Bradley DJ, Towle HC, Young WS. Spatial and temporal expression of alpha- and beta-thyroid hormone receptor mRNAs, including the beta 2-subtype, in the developing mammalian nervous system. J Neurosci Off J Soc Neurosci. 1992;12:2288–302.
8. Cheng SY. Multiple mechanisms for regulation of the transcriptional activity of thyroid hormone receptors. Rev Endocr Metab Disord. 2000;1:9–18.
9. Williams GR. Cloning and characterization of two novel thyroid hormone receptor beta isoforms. Mol Cell Biol. 2000;20:8329–42.
10. van der Spek AH, Fliers E, Boelen A. The classic pathways of thyroid hormone metabolism. Mol Cell Endocrinol. 2017;458:29–38.
11. Hammes SR, Davis PJ. Overlapping nongenomic and genomic actions of thyroid hormone and steroids. Best Pract Res Clin Endocrinol Metab. 2015;29:581–93.
12. Lin H-Y, Hopkins R, Cao HJ, Tang H-Y, Alexander C, Davis FB, et al. Acetylation of nuclear hormone receptor superfamily members: thyroid hormone causes acetylation of its own receptor by a mitogen-activated protein kinase-dependent mechanism. Steroids. 2005;70:444–9.
13. Davis PJ, Davis FB, Mousa SA, Luidens MK, Lin H-Y. Membrane receptor for thyroid hormone: physiologic and pharmacologic implications. Annu Rev Pharmacol Toxicol. 2011;51:99–115.
14. Bernal J. Thyroid hormones and brain development. Vitam Horm. 2005;71:95–122.
15. Berbel P, Ausó E, García-Velasco JV, Molina ML, Camacho M. Role of thyroid hormones in the maturation and organisation of rat barrel cortex. Neuroscience. 2001;107:383–94.
16. Aranda A, Pascual A. Nuclear hormone receptors and gene expression. Physiol Rev. 2001;81:1269–304.
17. Moog NK, Entringer S, Heim C, Wadhwa PD, Kathmann N, Buss C. Influence of maternal thyroid hormones during gestation on fetal brain development. Neuroscience. 2017;342:68–100.
18. Teixeira P de FDS, Dos Santos PB, Pazos-Moura CC. The role of thyroid hormone in metabolism and metabolic syndrome. Ther Adv Endocrinol Metab. 2020;11:2042018820917869.
19. Sinha RA, Singh BK, Yen PM. Direct effects of thyroid hormones on hepatic lipid metabolism. Nat Rev Endocrinol. 2018;14:259–69.
20. Bassett JHD, Williams GR. Role of thyroid hormones in skeletal development and bone maintenance. Endocr Rev. 2016;37:135–87.
21. Lazarus JH. Hyperthyroidism. Lancet Lond Engl. 1997;349:339–43.
22. Lazarus J, Obuobie K. Thyroid disorders—an update. Postgrad Med J. 2000;76:529–36.

# Hormones in Calcium Homeostasis

4

Manpreet Kaur and Kiran Prakash

**Abstract**

This chapter focuses on the hormones involved in homeostasis of calcium, namely vitamin D and parathyroid hormone (PTH). In the initial section—it discusses the details of biosynthesis, secretion and metabolism of vitamin D, followed by the mechanism of action of vitamin D, along with its clinical significance. Subsequently, there is an in-depth overview of PTH—the principal regulator of calcium levels in the body, including its biosynthesis, secretion, mechanism of action and associated clinical disorders.

**Keywords**

Homeostasis · Calcium · Vitamin D · Parathyroid hormone · Biosynthesis · Secretion · Mechanism of action · Applied aspects

Calcium and phosphate mineral homeostasis is critical for normal physiology. Moreover, calcium and phosphate are intricately inter-linked as both have an essential role in the formation of bone and teeth and have common players involved in their hormonal regulation and metabolism. The principal hormones involved in the regulation of calcium and phosphate balance are vitamin D and parathyroid hormone (PTH). This section describes in detail the physiology of these two hormones involved in mineral ion metabolism.

M. Kaur
Department of Physiology, VMMC and Safdarjung Hospital, New Delhi, India

K. Prakash (✉)
Department of Physiology, Government Medical College and Hospital, Sector 32, Chandigarh, India





H. Prabhakar, M. Kaur (eds.), *Brain and Endocrine Crosstalk*, Physiology in Clinical Neurosciences – Brain and Spinal Cord Crosstalks,
https://doi.org/10.1007/978-981-92-0763-3_4

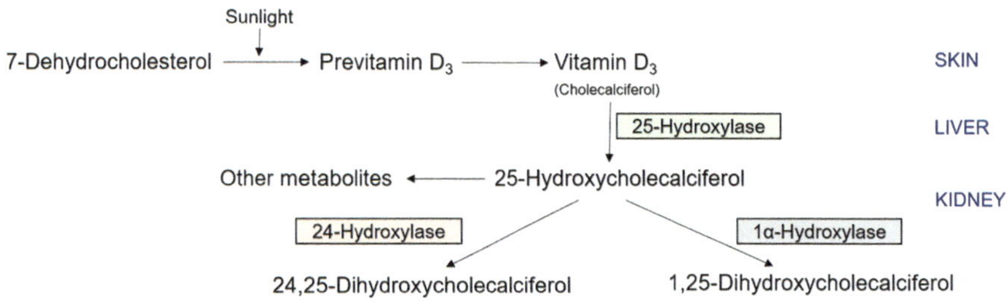


**Fig. 4.1** Successive steps involved in the formation of the physiologically active form (calcitriol) from vitamin D precursors. The formation of biologically active form vitamin D involves conversion at two levels—liver and kidney

## 4.1 Vitamin D

Vitamin D is involved in maintenance of a positive calcium balance and skeletal integrity.

### 4.1.1 Biosynthesis, Secretion and Metabolism of Vitamin D

Vitamin D comprises a group of closely related sterols (Fig. 4.1).

## 4.2 Primary Sources of Cholecalciferol: Skin and Diet

Vitamin $D_3$ (also called as cholecalciferol) is produced in the skin of mammals on exposure to sunlight from a precursor 7-dehydrocholesterol. This reaction involves initially the rapid formation of previtamin $D_3$ and then subsequent slower conversion to vitamin $D_3$. Therefore, adequate exposure to the Sun is known to prevent vitamin D deficiency. Some amount of vitamin $D_3$ is also directly ingested in the diet. Vitamin $D_3$ is further metabolized by enzymes in the liver and kidney.

## 4.3 Conversion of Cholecalciferol to 25-Hydroxycholecalciferol in the Liver

The first conversion occurs in the liver, where vitamin $D_3$ is converted to 25-hydroxycholecalciferol (also called as calcidiol or 25-(OH)$D_3$). This conversion step is limited because of the feedback inhibition of further conversion by the metabolite of this reaction that is 25-hydroxycholecalciferol itself. This feedback inhibition has some important implications.

1. The existence of this feedback mechanism regulates the concentration of 25-hydroxycholecalciferol in the plasma (although this step is not as tightly reg-

ulated as the subsequent 1α-hydroxylation step in the kidneys). Therefore, this somehow ensures that the concentration of 25-hydroxycholecalciferol remains nearly normal even when the dietary intake of vitamin $D_3$ has been increased several times. This acts as a protective mechanism preventing excess action of vitamin D due to dietary variations.

2. This controlled conversion of vitamin $D_3$ to 25-hydroxycholecalciferol aids in conserving and storing vitamin D effectively in the liver for future use. This is due to the fact that half-life of 25-hydroxycholecalciferol is only a few weeks, whereas in the form of vitamin $D_3$, it can be stored in the liver for many months.

The serum 25-hydroxycholecalciferol level is presently considered to be the best indicator of overall vitamin D status because its concentration reflects total body stores of vitamin D coming from both dietary intake and sunlight exposure, as well as other sources [1].

## 4.4 Further Conversion of 25-Hydroxycholecalciferol to the Biologically Active Form: 1,25-Dihydroxycholecalciferol in the Kidneys

25-Hydroxycholecalciferol is subsequently converted to the active metabolite 1,25-dihydroxycholecalciferol (also called as calcitriol or 1,25-$(OH)_2D_3$) in the cells of the proximal tubules of the kidneys. Calcitriol is also formed in other sites like the placenta, keratinocytes and macrophages. Nevertheless, some amount of 25-hydroxycholecalciferol is also converted to another less active metabolite 24,25-dihydroxycholecalciferol also in the kidney itself (Fig. 4.1) [2, 3].

### 4.4.1 Molecular Basis of Mechanism of Action

Vitamin D receptors (VDRs) are expressed by many cells of our body. These receptors have hormone binding and DNA binding domains. This further affects the transcriptional process and acts not only as a transcriptional activator for most genes but also as a transcriptional repressor in some cases [4].

### 4.4.2 Biological Actions of Vitamin D

The active form of vitamin D, that is calcitriol, acts principally on three organ systems of our body: the intestines, kidneys and bones. The net effect mediated by vitamin D is an increase in the absorption of calcium and phosphate into the extracellular fluid and hence contributes to the mineral ion homeostasis.

#### 4.4.2.1 Action on Intestine

Vitamin D increases the intestinal calcium transport across the enterocyte by augmenting all the three processes involved in calcium absorption (Fig. 4.2):

1. Increase the entry of calcium into the enterocyte

Vitamin D induces the expression of two major calcium transporters expressed by intestinal epithelia, TRPV5 and TRPV6 (transient receptor potential vanilloid), and also hastens its binding with the subjacent plasma membrane—calmodulin complex.

2. Increase in the transcellular transport of calcium

Vitamin D is a major inducer of calbindin 9K which is thought to play an important role in the transcellular transport of calcium across the enterocyte.

3. Exit from enterocyte to blood vessels

Basolateral plasma membrane calcium ATPases (PMCA1b isoform pump) gene of intestine is also vitamin D responsive. Its increased expression ensures the transport of absorbed calcium from intestine to extracellular fluid.

Vitamin D also promotes phosphate absorption by the intestines. It enhances the active transport of phosphate through the enterocyte by increasing the expression of

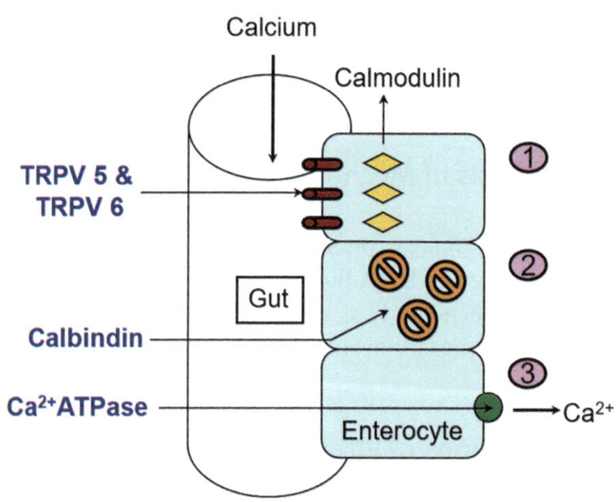


**Fig. 4.2** Steps involved in calcium transport across the intestinal enterocyte and the effect of vitamin D in augmenting the calcium flux. (1) Increase in calcium entry into the enterocyte by inducing the expression of calcium transporters in the apical membrane. (2) Increase in transcellular transport of calcium by calbindin. (3) Increase in basolateral transport of calcium by increased expression of vitamin D responsive calcium ATPase pump. *TRPV* transient receptor potential vanilloid

sodium-dependent phosphate cotransporters (NaPi-IIb isoform) and their insertion into enterocyte apical membrane [5–9].

#### 4.4.2.2 Action of Kidneys

Vitamin D increases the calcium and phosphate reabsorption by the epithelial cells of the renal tubules, thereby decreasing the renal calcium and phosphate excretion by mechanisms similar to intestine. It induces the expression of genes of apical calcium transporter (TRPV5 isoform), calbindin and the basolateral $Ca^{2+}$ ATPase (PMCA1b isoform) along with apical phosphate transporters, thereby resulting in increased calcium and phosphate reabsorption.

#### 4.4.2.3 Action on Bone

The VDR is expressed in osteoblasts and transcriptionally regulates the expression of several genes in this cell. Some genes are upregulated by calcitriol like the bone matrix proteins, osteocalcin and osteopontin, while others like type I collagen are repressed by calcitriol. This action predominates and promotes bone mineralization. Moreover, by its action on intestine and kidneys, it ensures adequate availability of calcium and phosphate for bone mineral deposition [10].

However, high doses of calcitriol also induce the expression of receptor activator of nuclear factor κ B (RANK) ligand. This action of calcitriol can cause bone resorption and is usually observed with higher doses of vitamin D (Fig. 4.3).

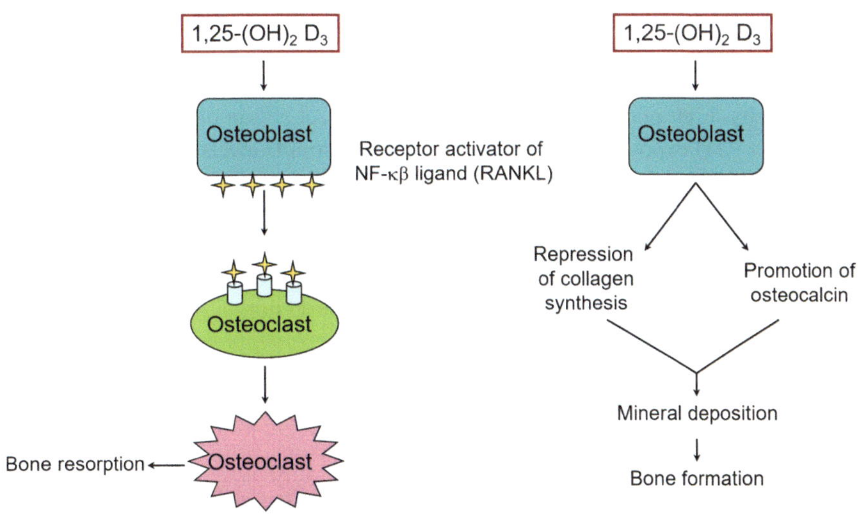


**Fig. 4.3** Actions of vitamin D on bone remodelling. Most importantly vitamin D is responsible for bone mineralization (as represented on the right side of the figure), while at extremely high doses, it can promote bone resorption as well

#### 4.4.2.4 Action on Parathyroid Gland

Calcitriol also regulates the gene transcription and cell proliferation in the parathyroid. Calcitriol directly inhibits PTH gene transcription and also stimulate the calcium-sensing receptor (CaSR) gene transcription [11].

## 4.5 Regulation of Vitamin D Metabolism

The levels of 25-hydroxycholecalciferol provide some amount of negative feedback to 25-hydroxylase. The 1α-hydroxylation step in kidneys is very tightly regulated and determines the availability of the active form of vitamin D—calcitriol. Upregulation of 1α-hydroxylase activity leads to increase in the active form of vitamin D. Calcitriol is responsible for most of the physiological actions of vitamin D (Fig. 4.4).

The following factors affect the balance of 1,25-dihydroxycholecalciferol (active form) to 24,25-dihydroxycholecalciferol (less active form) to have a controlled action of vitamin D [2, 3].

Calcium is one of the important regulators of vitamin D. When the plasma $Ca^{2+}$ level is high, a small amount of 1,25-dihydroxycholecalciferol (calcitriol) is produced. In addition, kidneys produce 24,25-dihydroxycholecalciferol instead, which has very low biological activity. This effect of $Ca^{2+}$ on production of 1,25-dihydroxycholecalciferol exerts its self-feedback, by further reducing the vitamin D-mediated $Ca^{2+}$ absorption from the intestine and thus bringing back the plasma calcium levels. In contrast, when the plasma $Ca^{2+}$ level is low, parathyroid hormone (PTH) secretion is increased, which in turn stimulates the expression of 1α-hydroxylase and thereby contributes to more action by the active metabolite of vitamin D.

Phosphate also plays a role in the regulation of vitamin D levels. Low plasma phosphate levels augment the production of 1,25-dihydroxycholecalciferol, while high phosphate levels have a direct inhibitory effect on the 1α-hydroxylase enzyme. Additionally, high phosphate levels also have a direct action on parathyroid gland and inhibit PTH expression and thus also affect vitamin D levels by determining the levels of PTH.

Fibroblast growth factor 23 (FGF23) has also been shown to repress the 1α-hydroxylase mRNA production and thus result in reduced levels of calcitriol.

Furthermore, the levels of vitamin D and the end-product of the reaction itself also exert a negative feedback control on further conversion.

### 4.5.1 Applied Aspects

#### 4.5.1.1 Vitamin D Deficiency

Clinical manifestation of vitamin D deficiency is called as rickets (in children) and osteomalacia (in adults). Rickets is characterized by growth retardation and expansion of growth plate. There are inadequate bone and teeth mineralization, and the bone mineral-to-matrix ratio is drastically reduced. Therefore, bones are fragile and

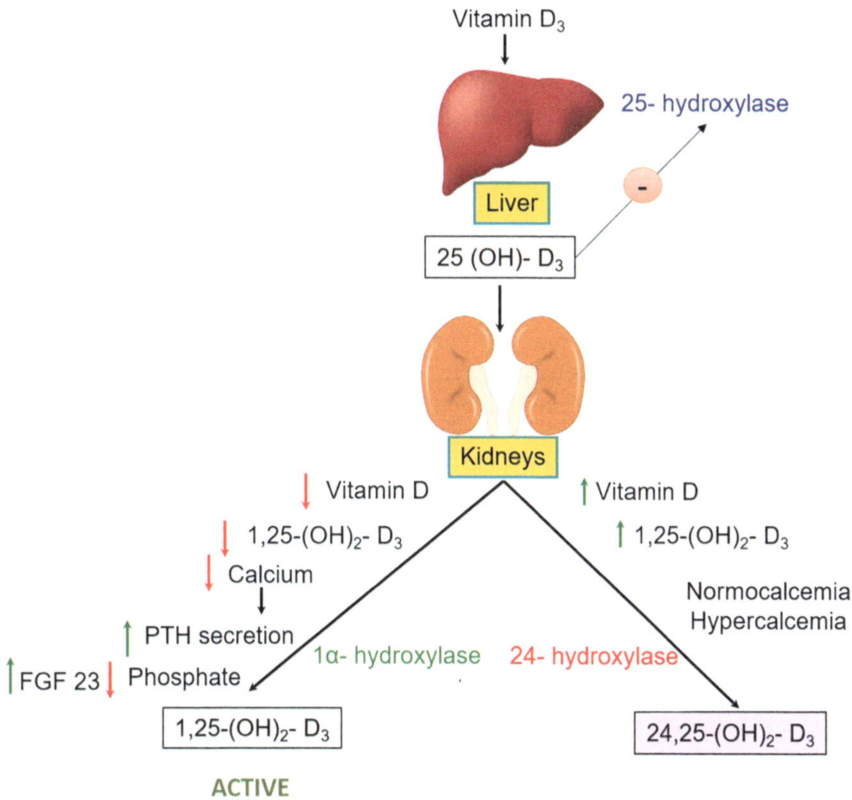


**Fig. 4.4** Regulation of vitamin D metabolism. Calcitriol (1,25-dihydroxycholecalciferol) levels are stringently maintained to meet the requirements of vitamin D by various regulatory factors—calcium (most important), phosphate, parathyroid hormone (PTH) and fibroblast growth factor 23 (FGF23). 24,25-dihydroxycholecalciferol is the less active form of vitamin D. Green arrows indicate increase, and red arrows signify decrease

prone to distortion when subjected to mechanical loads, resulting in bowing of weight-bearing joints (in children), severe bone pain and fractures [12, 13].

## 4.6 Parathyroid Hormone

The parathyroid hormone (PTH) is the principal hormone responsible for minute-to-minute maintenance of calcium ions in a relatively narrow range.

### 4.6.1 Biosynthesis, Secretion and Metabolism

Parathyroid hormone is the most important hormone responsible for maintaining extracellular fluid calcium concentration within a narrow normal range. Parathyroid gland cells have the ability to respond in multitudinous manner to adapt to the changing needs for PTH production in order to maintain calcium homeostasis. Firstly, there is a rapid release of the preformed hormone occurring within a few minutes in response to hypocalcaemia. This is followed by the second response that occurs within hours and involves the increased expression of PTH mRNA. Finally, after days of sustained stimulation, the parathyroid gland cells also have the potential to replicate to increase the mass of the gland.

PTH is synthesized as a larger precursor molecule which undergoes a series of cleavages to be finally converted to its active form (Fig. 4.5). It is initially synthesized as preproparathyroid hormone (115 amino acids), which undergoes cleavage to form proparathyroid hormone (90 amino acids) in the endoplasmic reticulum. Pre-sequence of gene has been shown to play a salient role in the hormone transport and secretion, while the role of the short pro-sequence has been speculated to help in the efficient working and accurate cleavage of the precursor sequence [14–16]. This is further secreted as the mature parathyroid hormone (84 amino acids) after removal of six amino acid residues from the amino terminal of proPTH in the Golgi apparatus and finally concentrated in the secretory vesicles and granules. The secretory granules also have few morphologically distinct subtypes which contain both PTH and the proteases cathepsin B and cathepsin H.

Regulation of biosynthetic steps (transcriptional and post-transcriptional) is an important mechanism to mediate changes in the available hormone levels in order to maintain calcium balance. PTH gene has near-maximal suppression of transcription at physiologic calcium concentrations. Transcriptional activity is increased within hours in response to hypocalcaemia. As mentioned earlier, calcitriol also

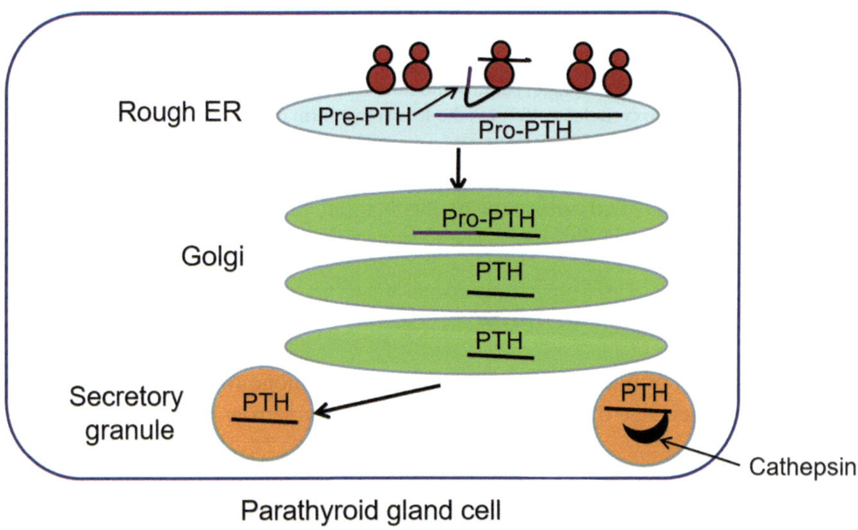


**Fig. 4.5** The steps of biosynthesis of parathyroid hormone. Prepro-PTH (115 amino acids) enters Golgi apparatus and is cleaved to pro-PTH (90 amino acids), which further processed to mature PTH (84 amino acids)

strongly suppresses the PTH gene transcription. Intracellular proteolytic degradation of newly synthesized PTH (posttranslational regulation of hormone production) is an important regulatory mechanism mediating the rapid changes in the hormone availability. For example, in conditions of hypercalcaemia, the secretion of PTH is substantially decreased, and most of secretion consists of the inactive carboxy-terminal fragments.

### 4.6.2 Molecular Basis of Mechanism of Action

Literature suggests the existence of three different G protein-coupled PTH receptors. The predominant one is the hPTH/PTHrP receptor, which also allows the parathyroid hormone-related protein (PTHrP) to bind to it. The second receptor is PTH2 (hPTH2-R) found in the brain, placenta and pancreas and does not bind to PTHrP. The hPTH/PTHrP receptor also activates the enzyme phospholipase C (PLC) via Gq subunit, thus resulting in an increase in intracellular calcium concentration and also activating the enzyme protein kinase C (Fig. 4.6) [17].

### 4.6.3 Biological Actions of PTH

PTH directly acts on kidney and bone, while an indirect action (mediated through vitamin D) on intestine, to finally contribute to maintenance of calcium equilibrium.

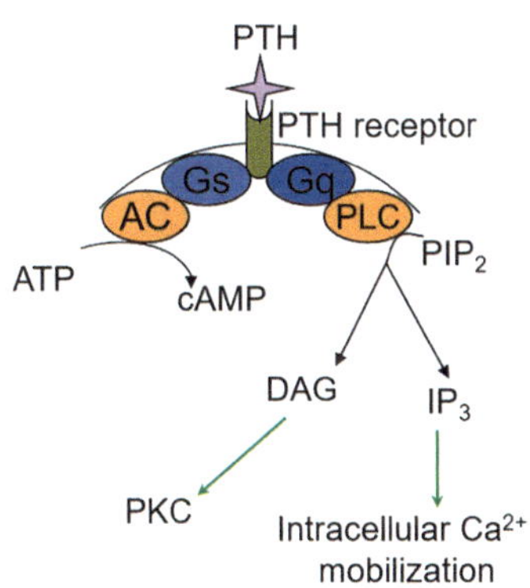


**Fig. 4.6** Molecular basis of parathyroid hormone (PTH) action. PTH binds to its G protein-coupled receptor to activate adenyl cyclase (AC) and phospholipase C (PLC) enzymes and lead to downstream signalling resulting in increase in intracellular cyclic AMP (cAMP), protein kinase C (PKC) activity and intracellular calcium concentration. *ATP* adenosine triphosphate, *AMP* adenosine monophosphate, $PIP_2$ phosphatidylinositol bisphosphate, *DAG* diacylglycerol, $IP_3$ inositol trisphosphate, $Ca^{2+}$ calcium

#### 4.6.3.1 Action on Kidney

Calcium reabsorption occurs in kidney by differing routes in different segments of renal tubules. PTH directly regulates the active, transcellular component, whereas the passive, paracellular route (which is primarily determined by the extent of concomitant sodium absorption) is indirectly affected by PTH. In the distal tubule, calcium absorption is entirely transcellular and is under regulation of PTH and calcitriol.

By increasing the activity of 1α-hydroxylase enzyme, it increases the availability of an active form of vitamin D that is calcitriol and also leads to calcitriol mediated increase in calcium absorption (as discussed above). Although, the major effects of PTH in calcium reabsorption are mediated through the transcellular route – it also effects the paracellular route by increasing the expression of paracellin-1 and $Na^+$ $K^+$ $2Cl^-$ cotransporter (Fig. 4.7) [17].

Phosphate absorption occurs via specific sodium-phosphate (NaPi) cotransporters, especially subtype IIa and subtype IIc. PTH causes the sequestration of these transporters within the subapical endocytic vesicles, and subsequently they undergo lysosomal degradation (Fig. 4.8) [18].

#### 4.6.3.2 Action on Bone

PTH action has complex manifestations on bone physiology as it acts on a number of bone cells either directly or indirectly. Stimulation of bone resorption to release calcium is the most prominent action of PTH on bone. However, PTH administration can also promote bone formation. Amongst them, which action dominates

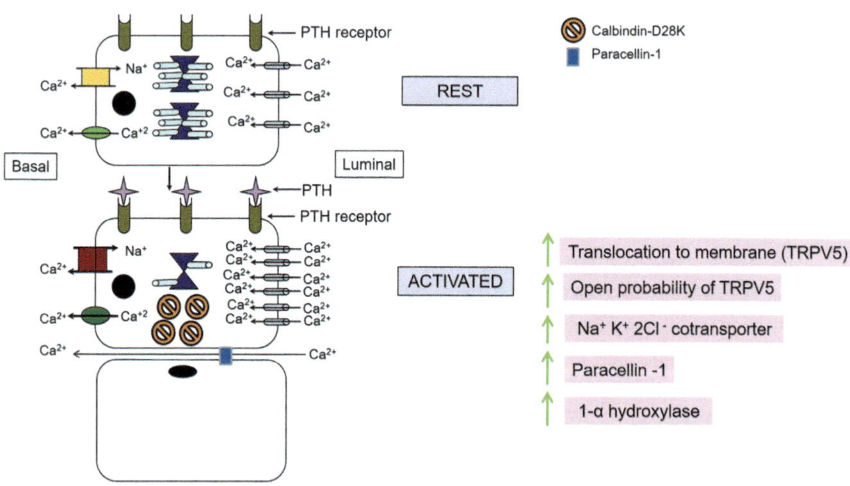


**Fig. 4.7** Action of parathyroid hormone (PTH) on calcium absorption in kidney. The upper panel depicts the basal state of renal epithelial cells with the machinery of calcium transport and PTH receptor. The lower panel shows the binding of PTH to its receptor resulting in increase in both paracellular route (by increase in expression of paracellin) and transcellular route (increasing the expression of proteins involved in calcium influx). *TRPV* transient receptor vanilloid, *$Ca^{2+}$* calcium, *$Na^+$* sodium

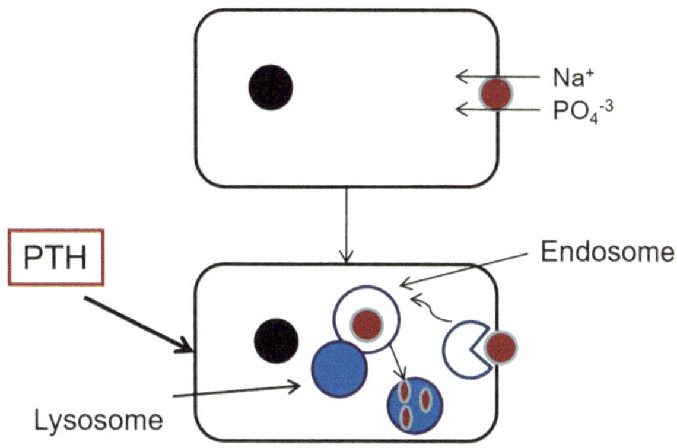


**Fig. 4.8** Action of parathyroid hormone (PTH) on phosphate absorption in kidney. PTH action causes the downregulation of sodium-phosphate transporter and hence causes increase in phosphate excretion by the kidney

depends on the dose and the route of administration of PTH. Continuous PTH administration results in bone resorption, decrease in bone mass and increase in blood calcium. On the contrary, intermittent administration of low doses of PTH leads to a net increase in bone mass. Mechanisms for these opposite effects of PTH are still not clear but have been speculated to be attributable to the action on different bone cell types, varying time course of these responses and the indirect autocrine and paracrine responses to PTH [19].

PTH causes an increase in calcium release from bone by augmenting two processes [20]:

- Rapid phase of calcium release by stimulating osteocytic osteolysis by increasing the calcium permeability of osteocyte membrane in contact with the bone fluid
- Slow phase of calcium release by stimulation of bone resorption by osteoclasts:
  - Promotes maturation of pro-osteoclasts to osteoclasts
  - Stimulates synthesis of lysosomal enzymes including collagenases and increase in release of acid by the osteoclasts
  - Increases the area of the resorptive zone of the osteoclasts

Although the most important action of PTH is considered to be bone resorption-the bone-resorbing cells that is osteoclasts, have no PTH receptors on their surfaces. Instead, PTH acts on the preosteoblasts and osteoblasts which in turn release secondary signals to the osteoclast precursors, to hasten the formation of mature osteoclasts and thus contribute to increase in number of osteoclasts. In addition, PTH signalling also augments the functional activity of mature osteoclasts to resorb bone and also prevents their apoptosis (Fig. 4.9).

Both macrophage colony stimulating factor (M-CSF) and receptor activator for nuclear factor κB ligand (RANKL) are essential for stimulation of the process of osteoclastogenesis [21]. Therefore, by all these mechanisms PTH results in increase in osteoclastic activity in a dual manner by increasing both the formation and activity of bone osteoclastic cells.

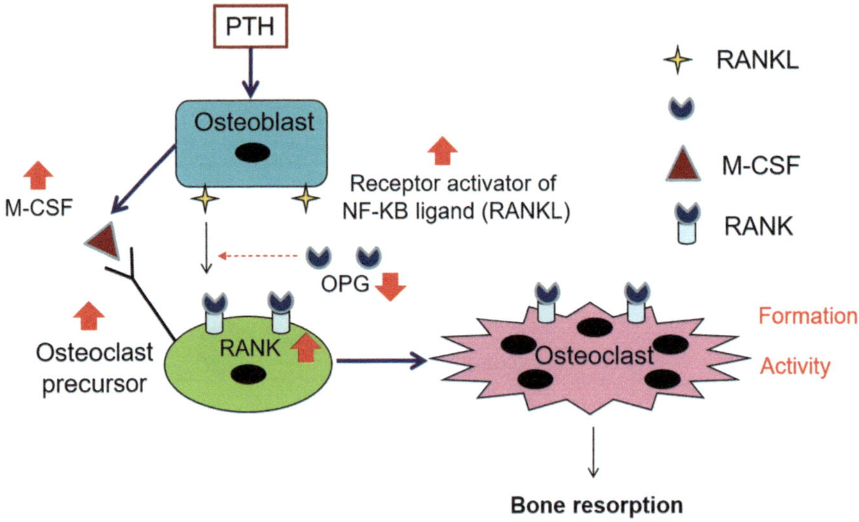


**Fig. 4.9** Action of parathyroid hormone (PTH) in bone. PTH acts on osteoblast cells and increases the expression of macrophage colony-stimulating factor (M-CSF) and receptor activator for nuclear factor κB ligand (RANKL) along with a decrease in osteoprotegerin (OPG). All these molecular signals culminate in an increase in both the formation and activity of mature osteoclasts, and resultant bone resorption

However, the action of intermittent PTH to increase bone formation by osteoblasts is probably an indirect one by autocrine and paracrine mediators. PTH causes release of growth factors such as insulin-like growth factor 1, fibroblast growth factor (FGF2) from osteoblastic cells [22]. These paracrine actions of PTH do not only stimulate the osteoblastic cells with PTH receptors but also activate, indirectly, the immature osteoblast precursors without PTH receptors. Furthermore, the process of bone resorption stimulated by PTH also releases osteoblast growth factors from bone matrix—which may also increase the osteoblastic activity and thus bone formation [23].

## 4.7 Overall Action of PTH on Plasma Calcium and Phosphate Levels

The net effect of PTH is an increase in plasma calcium levels and a decrease in plasma phosphate levels (Fig. 4.10).

### 4.7.1 Regulation of PTH

The regulation of parathyroid hormone (as mentioned above) occurs by two major mechanisms—regulation of PTH secretion and amplification of this regulation by intracellular degradation of stored hormone.

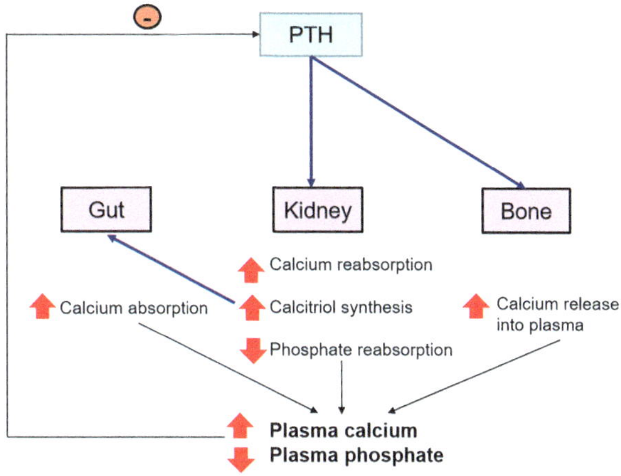


**Fig. 4.10** Overall action of parathyroid hormone (PTH) on plasma calcium and phosphate levels. PTH by its action on three organ systems—kidney, bone and intestine—finally mediates an effect of increase in plasma calcium levels with a decrease in plasma phosphate levels

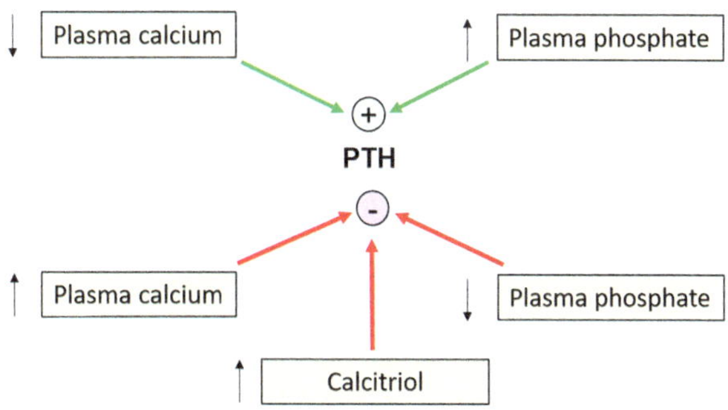


**Fig. 4.11** Regulation of parathyroid hormone (PTH). The important factors responsible for PTH regulation include plasma calcium, phosphate and calcitriol levels

The most important regulator is the concentration of ionized calcium in blood, although other stimuli—namely, phosphate, vitamin D and magnesium—also affect PTH secretion (Fig. 4.11).

#### 4.7.1.1 Calcium

Both synthesis and secretion of PTH are tightly controlled by a feedback system by the plasma ionized calcium concentrations. When the serum ionized calcium increases, there is a corresponding decrease in PTH secretion. The dose-response curve of calcium and PTH secretion is sigmoidal. This sigmoidal curve [24] has several important physiological implications:

- Minimal secretory rate of PTH is low, but not zero.
- Maximal secretory rate signifies the reserve of the parathyroid's capacity to respond to hypocalcaemia.
- Sensitivity represented by slope is maximal in the normal range of ionized calcium.

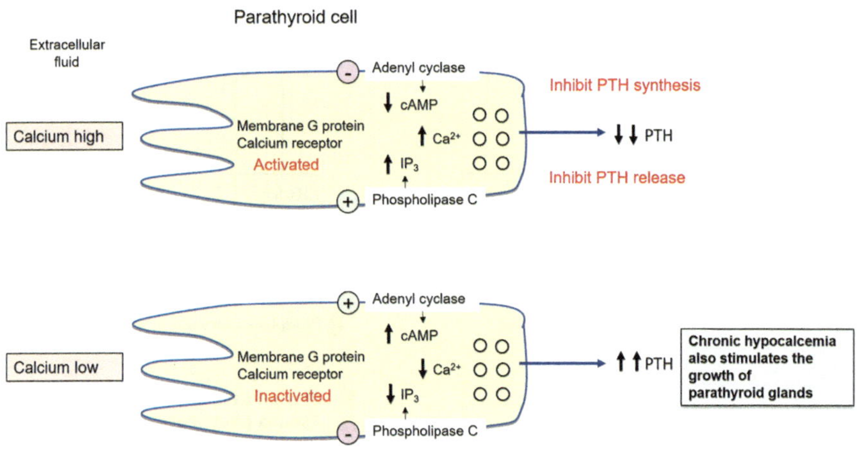


**Fig. 4.12** Regulation of parathyroid hormone (PTH) by plasma calcium. Plasma calcium levels are sensed by a membrane G protein-coupled calcium receptor which mediates further downstream signalling to modulate PTH synthesis and release

Studies have also shown that PTH secretion changes in response to both the absolute levels and the rate of change in the ionized calcium levels. This property provides an additional protection against episodes of sudden hypocalcaemia.

The changes in plasma ionized calcium levels are detected by a special plasma membrane receptor known as parathyroid calcium sensing receptor (CaSR) [25]. This activity stimulates the release of calcium from intracellular stores, which, in turn, feedbacks to decrease the PTH secretion (Fig. 4.12).

Moreover, different studies have also suggested the underlying mechanism for the increase in PTH mRNA in response to hypocalcaemia from regulation at the levels of gene transcription, mRNA translation to mRNA stability.

#### 4.7.1.2 Vitamin D

Calcitriol directly suppresses PTH gene transcription by inhibiting the synthesis of the prepro-PTH mRNA [26]. Interestingly, this transcriptional suppression is not observed when calcitriol is administered in conditions of chronic hypocalcaemia, probably because hypocalcaemia leads to a fall in the number of parathyroid cell vitamin D receptors (VDRs) or because hypocalcaemia leads to increase in the expression of calreticulin in the parathyroid [27].

#### 4.7.1.3 Phosphate

Phosphate can directly stimulate PTH synthesis and indirectly stimulates the PTH synthesis and release by reducing ionic calcium levels and also by mediating a decrease in calcitriol levels [28].

### 4.7.2 Parathyroid Hormone-Related Protein (PTHrP)

PTHrP was discovered because of its secretion by a variety of tumours with a manifestation of humoral hypercalcaemia of malignancy. Studies suggested the structural homology of PTHrP to PTH, thereby allowing it to act on hPTH/PTHrP receptor and mimic the physiologic effects of PTH in bone and kidney. However, recent literature indicates that normally also PTHrP, unlike PTH, is made by a wide variety of tissues and acts locally to bring about different actions. However, it is not involved in calcium homeostasis [13].

Table 4.1 below compares and contrasts some of the important facts regarding the two—PTH and PTHrP.

### 4.7.3 Applied Aspects

Some of the disorders associated with PTH hormone or disbalance in calcium homeostasis are discussed below [12, 13].

#### 4.7.3.1 Primary Hyperparathyroidism

Excess PTH production is often due to parathyroid gland hyperplasia, adenoma or carcinoma. It is characterized by the presence of elevated intact PTH levels, hypercalcaemia, hypercalciuria with increased formation of kidney stones (urolithiasis)

**Table 4.1** Comparison of parathyroid hormone (PTH) and parathyroid hormone related protein (PTHrP)

| Parameter | PTH | PTHrP |
|---|---|---|
| Action | Endocrine | Paracrine |
| Sites | Predominantly parathyroid glands | Skin, hair, breast and few other sites |
| Functions | Calcium phosphate homeostasis, vitamin D activation, bone remodelling | Regulate proliferation and differentiation, relaxation of smooth muscle to stretch in blood vessels, bladder and uterus. During lactation, promotes bone resorption and transport of calcium to milk. During development, calcium transport across placenta and key regulator of chondrocyte proliferation and differentiation in growth plates of long bones |
| Regulation | Primarily calcium | Not by calcium |
| Structure | 84 amino acids | 140 amino acids (30 AA homology at N terminal) |
| Gene | Chromosome 12 | Chromosome 11 |

and decreased plasma phosphate levels. Characteristic clinical features include abdominal groans (constipation, nausea, vomiting and peptic ulcer), bones (osteitis fibrosa with subperiosteal resorption, osteoclastomas and bone cysts, radiological findings of osteoporosis/rickets/osteomalacia and arthritis), stones (renal stones) and psychic moans (lethargy, fatigue, depression, paranoia and personality changes).

#### 4.7.3.2 Secondary Hyperparathyroidism

They comprise disorders where the excess PTH production is due to a manifestation of disorders that do not affect the parathyroid gland primarily rather a response to hypocalcaemia. The most common disorder in this category is the condition of chronic renal failure. As calcitriol (active form of vitamin D) is formed in the kidney, there is reduction in plasma calcitriol and subsequently a moderate fall in ionized calcium, which contributes to a greater synthesis and secretion of PTH.

#### 4.7.3.3 Humoral Hypercalcaemia of Malignancy

These include cancers of skin, breast and others which ectopically synthesize excess PTHrP which mimics the action of PTH and thus manifest hypercalcaemia.

#### 4.7.3.4 Primary Hypoparathyroidism

They are commonly associated with other endocrine disorders and neoplasia or may result from inadvertent surgical removal of the parathyroid glands during thyroid surgery. The patient characteristically presents with hypocalcaemic tetany. Amongst the muscles of the body, laryngeal muscles are most prone to spasm. Spasm of these muscles could be life-threatening as they obstruct respiration and needs to be taken care immediately.

#### 4.7.3.5 Pseudohypoparathyroidism

This is characterized by a PTH receptor defect, and therefore the patient presents with the signs and symptoms of hypoparathyroidism, although circulating PTH levels are either normal or elevated.

#### 4.7.3.6 Familial Hypercalciuric Hypocalcaemia

This is characterized by a gain of function mutation in calcium receptor gene which leads to an increase in sensitivity of negative feedback resulting in decrease in PTH, and hence hypocalcaemia is observed.

## References

1. Heaney RP. The vitamin D requirement in health and disease. J Steroid Biochem Mol Biol. 2005;97(1–2):13–9.
2. Jones G, Strugnell SA, DeLuca HF. Current understanding of the molecular actions of vitamin D. Physiol Rev. 1998;78(4):1193–231.
3. Bikle D. Vitamin D: production, metabolism, and mechanisms of action. In: Feingold KR, Anawalt B, Boyce A, Chrousos G, Dungan K, Grossman A, et al., editors. Endotext [Internet].

South Dartmouth: MDText.com, Inc.; 2000 [cited 2020 July 3]. Available from: http://www.ncbi.nlm.nih.gov/books/NBK278935/.

4. Inoue T, Kamiyama J, Sakai T. Sp1 and NF-Y synergistically mediate the effect of vitamin D(3) in the p27(Kip1) gene promoter that lacks vitamin D response elements. J Biol Chem. 1999;274(45):32309–17.
5. Karbach U. Paracellular calcium transport across the small intestine. J Nutr. 1992;122(3 Suppl):672–7.
6. Fujita H, Sugimoto K, Inatomi S, Maeda T, Osanai M, Uchiyama Y, et al. Tight junction proteins claudin-2 and -12 are critical for vitamin D-dependent Ca2+ absorption between enterocytes. Mol Biol Cell. 2008;19(5):1912–21.
7. van de Graaf SFJ, Boullart I, Hoenderop JGJ, Bindels RJM. Regulation of the epithelial Ca2+ channels TRPV5 and TRPV6 by 1alpha,25-dihydroxy vitamin D3 and dietary Ca2+. J Steroid Biochem Mol Biol. 2004;89–90(1–5):303–8.
8. Hoenderop JGJ, van Leeuwen JPTM, van der Eerden BCJ, Kersten FFJ, van der Kemp AWCM, Mérillat A-M, et al. Renal Ca2+ wasting, hyperabsorption, and reduced bone thickness in mice lacking TRPV5. J Clin Invest. 2003;112(12):1906–14.
9. Benn BS, Ajibade D, Porta A, Dhawan P, Hediger M, Peng J-B, et al. Active intestinal calcium transport in the absence of transient receptor potential vanilloid type 6 and calbindin-D9k. Endocrinology. 2008;149(6):3196–205.
10. Yasuda H, Shima N, Nakagawa N, Yamaguchi K, Kinosaki M, Mochizuki S, et al. Osteoclast differentiation factor is a ligand for osteoprotegerin/osteoclastogenesis-inhibitory factor and is identical to TRANCE/RANKL. Proc Natl Acad Sci USA. 1998;95(7):3597–602.
11. Meir T, Levi R, Lieben L, Libutti S, Carmeliet G, Bouillon R, et al. Deletion of the vitamin D receptor specifically in the parathyroid demonstrates a limited role for the receptor in parathyroid physiology. Am J Physiol Renal Physiol. 2009;297(5):F1192–8.
12. Jameson JL. Chapter 25, Bone and mineral metabolism in health and disease. In: Harrison's endocrinology. 2nd ed. New York: The McGraw-Hill Companies; 2010. p. 388–405.
13. Melmed S, Polonsky KS, Larsen PR, Kronenberg HM. Chapter 28, Hormones and disorders of mineral metabolism. In: William's textbook of endocrinology. 12th ed. Philadelphia: Elsevier Saunders; 2011. p. 1237–304.
14. Arnold A, Horst SA, Gardella TJ, Baba H, Levine MA, Kronenberg HM. Mutation of the signal peptide-encoding region of the preproparathyroid hormone gene in familial isolated hypoparathyroidism. J Clin Invest. 1990;86(4):1084–7.
15. Sunthornthepvarakul T, Churesigaew S, Ngowngarmratana S. A novel mutation of the signal peptide of the preproparathyroid hormone gene associated with autosomal recessive familial isolated hypoparathyroidism. J Clin Endocrinol Metab. 1999;84(10):3792–6.
16. Wiren KM, Potts JT, Kronenberg HM. Importance of the propeptide sequence of human preproparathyroid hormone for signal sequence function. J Biol Chem. 1988;263(36):19771–7.
17. Reilly RF, Ellison DH. Mammalian distal tubule: physiology, pathophysiology, and molecular anatomy. Physiol Rev. 2000;80(1):277–313.
18. Segawa H, Yamanaka S, Onitsuka A, Tomoe Y, Kuwahata M, Ito M, et al. Parathyroid hormone-dependent endocytosis of renal type IIc Na-Pi cotransporter. Am J Physiol Renal Physiol. 2007;292(1):F395–403.
19. Jilka RL. Molecular and cellular mechanisms of the anabolic effect of intermittent PTH. Bone. 2007;40(6):1434–46.
20. Datta NS, Abou-Samra AB. PTH and PTHrP signaling in osteoblasts. Cell Signal. 2009;21(8):1245–54.
21. Teitelbaum SL, Ross FP. Genetic regulation of osteoclast development and function. Nat Rev Genet. 2003;4(8):638–49.
22. Qin L, Tamasi J, Raggatt L, Li X, Feyen JHM, Lee DC, et al. Amphiregulin is a novel growth factor involved in normal bone development and in the cellular response to parathyroid hormone stimulation. J Biol Chem. 2005;280(5):3974–81.
23. Tang Y, Wu X, Lei W, Pang L, Wan C, Shi Z, et al. TGF-beta1-induced migration of bone mesenchymal stem cells couples bone resorption with formation. Nat Med. 2009;15(7):757–65.

24. Parfitt AM. New concepts of bone remodeling: a unified spatial and temporal model with physiologic and pathophysiologic implications. In: Agarwal SC, Stout SD, editors. Bone loss and osteoporosis: an anthropological perspective [Internet]. Boston: Springer US; 2003 [cited 2020 July 14]. p. 3–17. Available from: https://doi.org/10.1007/978-1-4419-8891-1_1.
25. Hofer AM, Brown EM. Extracellular calcium sensing and signalling. Nat Rev Mol Cell Biol. 2003;4(7):530–8.
26. Silver J, Naveh-Many T, Mayer H, Schmelzer HJ, Popovtzer MM. Regulation by vitamin D metabolites of parathyroid hormone gene transcription in vivo in the rat. J Clin Invest. 1986;78(5):1296–301.
27. Sela-Brown A, Russell J, Koszewski NJ, Michalak M, Naveh-Many T, Silver J. Calreticulin inhibits vitamin D's action on the PTH gene in vitro and may prevent vitamin D's effect in vivo in hypocalcemic rats. Mol Endocrinol Baltim Md. 1998;12(8):1193–200.
28. Kilav R, Silver J, Naveh-Many T. Parathyroid hormone gene expression in hypophosphatemic rats. J Clin Invest. 1995;96(1):327–33.

# Adrenal Gland

# 5

Manpreet Kaur

**Abstract**

The adrenal gland is an essential endocrine organ comprising two parts—adrenal cortex and adrenal medulla. The adrenal cortex secretes three categories of hormones—mineralocorticoids, glucocorticoids and adrenal androgens. This chapter focuses on the biosynthesis, metabolism, mechanism of action, regulation and disorders of these hormones. The understanding of these concepts is essential for clinical diagnosis and management of various endocrine disorders.

**Keywords**

Mineralocorticoids · Glucocorticoids · Sex hormones · Biosynthesis · Metabolism · Biological actions · Regulation · Applied aspects

## 5.1 Adrenal Hormones: Mineralocorticoids, Glucocorticoids and Sex Hormones

Adrenal gland is an important gland of the endocrine system with components of two different embryological origins. The two adrenal glands are situated on the top of each kidney (Fig. 5.1). The outer adrenal cortex (90% of the weight of the adrenals) is derived from mesodermal tissue, while the inner medulla (10% of the weight of adrenals) is derived from neural crest cells.

The three layers of adrenal cortex as well as the adrenal medulla have characteristic morphological features and enzymatic specificities and hence secrete specific hormones. These hormones in turn have distinct physiological actions and key regulators (Table 5.1).

M. Kaur (✉)
Department of Physiology, VMMC and Safdarjung Hospital, New Delhi, India





H. Prabhakar, M. Kaur (eds.), *Brain and Endocrine Crosstalk*, Physiology in Clinical Neurosciences – Brain and Spinal Cord Crosstalks,
https://doi.org/10.1007/978-981-92-0763-3_5

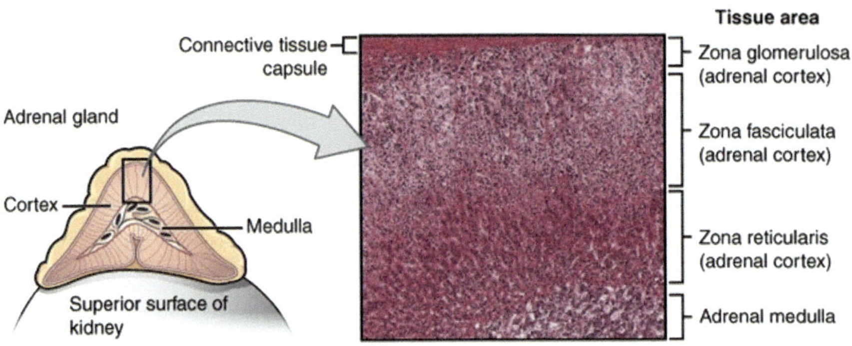


**Fig. 5.1** The structure of adrenal cortex and medulla. The cortex is further divided into three zones that have distinct enzymatic capacities, leading to a relative specificity in the products of each of the adrenal cortex zones (available at https://commons.wikimedia.org/wiki/File:1818_The_Adrenal_Glands.jpg)

**Table 5.1** Hormones of adrenal gland—their site of secretion and key physiological regulators

| Layers (weight) | | Hormone production | Main regulators |
|---|---|---|---|
| Cortex (72%) | Zona glomerulosa (15%) | Mineralocorticoids:<br>Aldosterone (main)<br>Deoxycorticosterone | Ang II (main)<br>Potassium<br>ACTH |
| | Zona fasciculata (50%) | Glucocorticoids (main)<br>(a) Cortisol<br>(b) Cortisone<br>Sex steroids | ACTH |
| | Zona reticularis (7%) | Sex steroids (main)<br>(a) Dehydroepiandrosterone<br>(b) Androstenedione<br>Glucocorticoids | ACTH |
| Medulla (28%) | | Epinephrine (90%)<br>Norepinephrine (10%) | Sympathetic system |

## 5.2 Hormones of the Adrenal Cortex

The adrenal cortical hormones derive their name by the principal action performed by them. Mineralocorticoids are essential for the maintenance of sodium balance and extracellular fluid (ECF) volume. Glucocorticoids predominantly affect metabolism of carbohydrate and protein.

### 5.2.1 Biosynthesis of Adrenal Steroid Hormones

All the hormones of the adrenal cortex are derived from cholesterol and hence contain the cyclopentanoperhydrophenanthrene ring. Cholesterol from the diet and endogenous synthesis is the substrate for steroidogenesis [1]. The existence of the

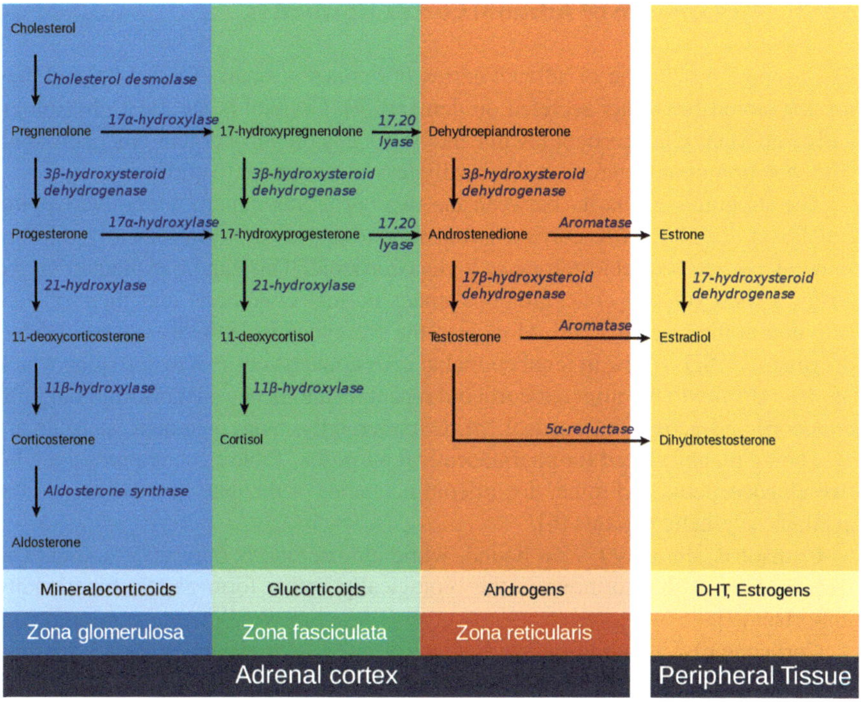


**Fig. 5.2** The major pathways of adrenal steroid biosynthesis. (Available at https://en.wikipedia.org/wiki/Adrenal_cortex)

three major adrenal biosynthetic pathways leads to the production of specific hormones by the separate zones of the adrenal cortex [2] (Fig. 5.2).

## 5.3 Genetic Defects in Biosynthetic Enzymes of Adrenal Steroids

Inherited genetic defects can cause relative or absolute deficiencies in the biosynthetic enzymes involved in steroidogenesis [3]. Most commonly encountered are those that affect the steroidogenic enzymes required for the formation of cortisol. Thus, these disorders are collectively termed as congenital adrenal hypertrophy.

Among them, the most common is mutation of 21-hydroxylase which impairs the formation of cortisol, corticosterone and aldosterone. Because of reduction in these hormones, ACTH secretion is increased resulting in hypertrophy of adrenal glands and increased conversion of pregnenolone to adrenal androgens. Consequently, women with this defect manifest virilization.

### 5.3.1 Metabolism of Adrenal Cortex Hormones

The average production of adrenal cortex hormones is small (Table 5.2), and they are not stored but rather secreted on demand [4]. Cortisol is the most physiologically important glucocorticoid, while aldosterone is the most potent glucocorticoid. The secretion of aldosterone is drastically less as compared to cortisol.

The structural similarity between the two corticoids imparts them overlapping functional abilities. Still, cortisol is not functioning as a physiologically relevant mineralocorticoid or aldosterone as a glucocorticoid. This can be explained on the basis of their relative concentrations under normal conditions and their relative activities at the receptor level. Moreover, the presence of 11β-hydroxysteroid dehydrogenase (HSD) type 2 in renal epithelial cells converts cortisol to cortisone which has less affinity to the mineralocorticoid receptors and hence ensures minimal mineralocorticoid activity of cortisol [5]. Commercially, many synthetic steroids are also being manufactured for pharmaceutical purposes. Table 5.3 compares the relative glucocorticoid and mineralocorticoid potencies of the natural analogues to the available synthetic variants [6].

Cortisol is almost 90–95% bound, while aldosterone is only 60% bound. The free fraction of the hormone is the biologically active form and is functionally important [7].

Consequently, in conditions with altered synthesis of plasma proteins, the total cortisol might change. For example, during pregnancy placental production of oestrogen stimulates synthesis of plasma proteins by liver. When plasma protein levels fall in cirrhosis, nephrosis, and multiple myeloma, the opposite is observed, resulting in a decrease in total cortisol levels.

**Table 5.2** Average daily production of adrenal cortex hormones

| Hormone | Amount (mg/day) |
|---|---|
| Cortisol | 20 |
| Corticosterone | 2 |
| Aldosterone | 0.1 |
| Dehydroepiandrosterone | 30 |

**Table 5.3** Comparison of glucocorticoid and mineralocorticoid activities of various steroids (as compared to cortisol)

| Steroid | Glucocorticoid activity | Mineralocorticoid activity |
|---|---|---|
| Cortisol | 1 | 1 |
| Corticosterone | 0.3 | 15 |
| Aldosterone | 0.3 | 3000 |
| Deoxycorticosterone | 0.2 | 100 |
| Prednisolone | 4 | 0.8 |
| Fluorocortisol | 10 | 125 |
| Dexamethasone | 25 | 0 |

Adrenal steroid hormones are catabolized primarily by the liver to be excreted in the urine. They are eliminated principally in the form of metabolites like tetrahydrocortisol glucuronide and 17-ketosteroids analogues [8]. The unconjugated form of etiocholanolone can cause fever when it is unconjugated. Some amount of aldosterone is converted in the liver and kidneys to an 18-glucuronide.

## 5.3.2 Biological Actions and Underlying Molecular Mechanism of Adrenal Cortical Hormones

### 5.3.2.1 Mineralocorticoids

#### Cellular Mechanism of Action

They have been shown to have both rapid (non-genomic) and gradual (genomic) actions [9, 10].

#### Genomic Action

The mineralocorticoids are lipid soluble and rapidly diffuse to interior of renal epithelial cells. Although MR receptors in renal tubular epithelial cells have a high affinity for cortisol (which is present in higher concentrations), the enzyme 11β-hydroxysteroid dehydrogenase type 2 (HSD2) converts most of the cortisol to cortisone, which lacks affinity for MR receptors (as discussed above). Then this aldosterone-receptor complex diffuses into the nucleus and finally causes transcriptional changes in gene expression. Therefore, the peak effect of aldosterone is only manifested after several hours as the genomic effects require gene transcription and synthesis of new protein and thus have a latency of 45–60 min.

#### Non-genomic Action

Some studies report also a faster action within seconds to minutes, mediated by binding to cell membrane receptors that are coupled to second messenger systems. The generation of cyclic adenosine monophosphate (cAMP) in vascular smooth muscle cells and in epithelial cells of the renal collecting tubules occurs in less than 2 minutes, a period far too short for gene transcription and the synthesis of new proteins.

#### Biological Action

They principally affect the function of two cell types—epithelial and non-epithelial.

##### Epithelial Cells

The major function of mineralocorticoids (most importantly aldosterone) is the regulation of extracellular fluid volume and potassium homeostasis [11]. Aldosterone binds to mineralocorticoid receptors in epithelial cells, primarily the principal cells in the renal cortical collecting duct. Through the genomic action of aldosterone, it increases not only the number but also activity of all three channels (epithelial sodium channels, the sodium-potassium pump and the potassium selective luminal channels) involved in reabsorption of sodium and excretion of potassium (Fig. 5.3). Water accompanies the absorbed sodium, therefore increasing the blood volume. As the concentration of hydrogen ion is also greater in the lumen than in the cell, hydrogen ion is also actively secreted. A similar action of mineralocorticoids is observed in epithelial cells at other sites, namely salivary ducts, sweat glands and gastrointestinal tract to cause reabsorption of sodium in exchange for potassium.

There exists a noteworthy phenomenon of 'aldosterone escape'. When normal individuals are given aldosterone, there is an initial period of sodium retention, which is followed by natriuresis. As a consequence, oedema does not develop in them. The underlying mechanism of this escape is dual. Firstly, volume expansion by excess sodium and water causes an increase in glomerular filtration rate (GFR), which increases the sodium delivery to the distal nephron. This increased delivery of sodium ($Na^+$) overrides the enhanced aldosterone-mediated $Na^+$ reabsorption. This leads to excretion of both $Na^+$ and water (pressure natriuresis and diuresis). Secondly, volume expansion also culminates to an increase in plasma atrial natriuretic peptide (ANP) which in turn has natriuretic action. However, it is important to remember that there is no such escape from the potassium-losing effects of mineralocorticoids.

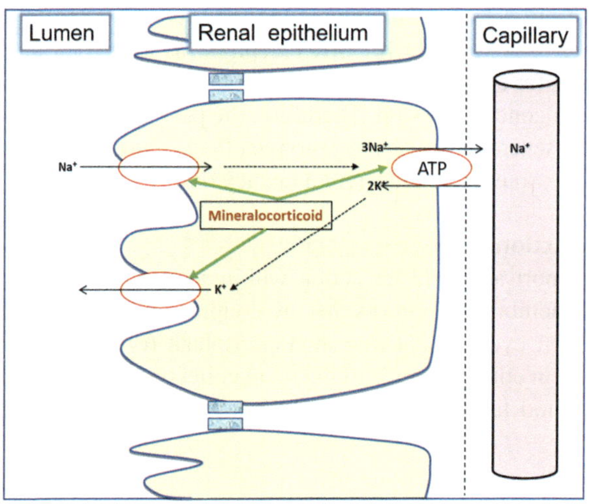


**Fig. 5.3** Action of mineralocorticoids on renal epithelial cells of collecting ducts. Sodium moves passively through epithelial sodium channels on apical membrane of renal epithelial cells down their electrochemical gradient. This is then actively extruded from the basolateral side by the sodium-potassium pump. This active pump also provides the necessary driving force for pushing potassium into the urine through potassium selective luminal channels again along its electrochemical gradient. Mineralocorticoids facilitate all the three activities and hence promote sodium retention at the cost of potassium loss

Non-epithelial Cells

Mineralocorticoid receptors are also present on some non-epithelial cells like neurons, myocytes, endothelial cells and vascular smooth muscle cells. The action at these sites differs from the epithelial cells in the following manner [11, 12]:

(a) They do not affect the sodium-potassium homeostasis.
(b) The group of genes regulated at these sites is different. For example, here it modulates the expression of genes involved in tissue growth factors, e.g., transforming growth factor (TGF) β, adiponectin and leptin, to name a few.
(c) 11-HSD 2 enzyme expression may differ, and hence the deactivation of cortisol would depend on this enzyme expression. At some sites (e.g., myocardium and brain), the enzyme is deficient, and hence the mineralocorticoid receptor is not protected and cortisol rather than aldosterone acts on it. Furthermore, in other tissues (e.g., the vasculature), 11-HSD 2 is expressed in a manner similar to the epithelial cells, and therefore the predominant action of aldosterone occurs on the mineralocorticoid receptor.
(d) Some of the manifestations of aldosterone are very rapid and thus via its non-genomic action. They are considered to be secondary to the activation of a cell surface receptor.
(e) Some of these cells like the myocardium and vasculature may locally produce some aldosterone, although this theory is still controversial.

#### 5.3.2.2 Glucocorticoids

##### Cellular Mechanism of Action

Glucocorticoids bind to the α subunit of glucocorticoid receptors (GRs) in the cytosol and result in the activation of the steroid-receptor complex through a process that involves the dissociation of heat shock proteins [13]. Subsequently, this complex is translocated to the nucleus, where they bind to a specific DNA sequence in the promoter region of certain target genes termed as glucocorticoid-response element (GRE). There on the transcription of the certain genes is stimulated or repressed [14]. Like with mineralocorticoids, non-genomic effects due to binding to some uncharacterized membrane-coupled receptors bringing about rapid (within seconds or minutes) have also been reported for glucocorticoids [10].

##### Biological Actions

1. Carbohydrate, Protein and Lipid Metabolism

The net effect of glucocorticoids on the intermediary metabolism of carbohydrate, protein and lipid is to increase blood glucose concentration. This provides the essential fuel glucose to vital organs (brain and heart) in states of increase requirement like stress (Fig. 5.4).

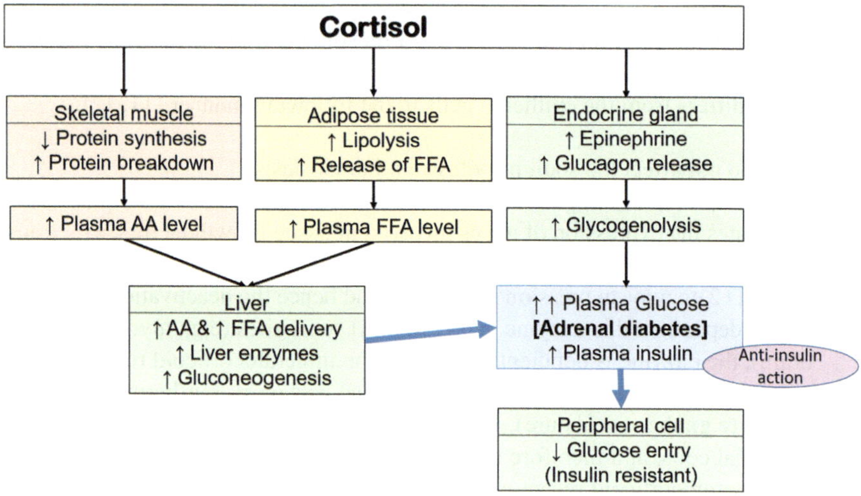


**Fig. 5.4** Effect of glucocorticoids on the carbohydrate, protein and lipid metabolism

## Carbohydrate Metabolism

(a) *Stimulation of gluconeogenesis.* Corticosteroids increase the rate of gluconeogenesis (i.e., formation of glucose from other sources) by almost six- to tenfold. This metabolic effect is mainly attributable due to the following actions of glucocorticoids:

1. They increase the transcription of enzymes involved in gluconeogenesis in liver cells [15].
2. They cause mobilization of amino acids (additional source for gluconeogenesis) from the extrahepatic tissues, mainly from muscle.
3. They antagonize inhibitory effect of insulin on gluconeogenesis in the liver.

Therefore, overall effect of glucocorticoids is to increase the glucose output by the liver. Moreover, the increase in glycogen storage in liver cells that accompanies increased gluconeogenesis potentiates the effects of other glycolytic hormones, such as epinephrine and glucagon, to mobilize glucose in times of need, such as between meals (permissive role).

(b) *Decreased glucose utilization by cells.* Glucocorticoids cause a moderate decrease in glucose utilization by most cells in the body [16]. They cause a decrease in translocation of the glucose transporters GLUT 4 to the cell membrane, especially in skeletal muscle cells, leading to insulin resistance. Also, glucocorticoids reduce the expression of insulin receptor substrate-1 and phosphatidylinositol 3 kinase, both of which are involved in mediating the actions of insulin, as well as oxidation of nicotinamide-adenine dinucleotide (NADH) to form $NAD^+$. NADH must be oxidized for the process of glycolysis, thus again resulting in decrease in the usage of glucose by cells.

(c) *Adrenal diabetes.* Glucocorticoids increase the rate of production of glucose and also reduce the rate of utilization at the same time and therefore cause a drastic increase in blood glucose concentration. This in turn is a potent stimulus for the release of insulin. However, functionally this insulin is ineffective in maintaining plasma glucose levels. As discussed above, excess glucocorticoids result in a situation of insulin resistance, especially in skeletal muscle and adipose tissue. Moreover, glucocorticoids effect the expression of glucose transporters and enzymes involved in glucose regulation and also the high levels of fatty acid accumulation together further impair the actions of insulin on the tissues. In this manner, the increase in glucocorticoids produces disturbances in carbohydrate metabolism that mimics clinical condition with growth hormone excess. This condition with an increase in blood glucose concentration is insensitive to the administration of insulin and is called as adrenal diabetes.

**Protein Metabolism**

Glucocorticoids reduce the total protein content in essentially all cells of the body (except the liver).

(a) *Reduction in cellular protein.* The decrease in the protein stores is observed due to both a fall in protein synthesis and increased breakdown in the cells. These effects may partly be seen due to the reduced amino acid transport to the extrahepatic tissues, especially in muscle and lymphoid tissue. Due to this reason, patients with elevated glucocorticoids experience extreme muscle weakness and immune deficiency manifestations.

(b) *Increase in liver and plasma proteins.* Interestingly, liver proteins are an exception to the protein depleting effect of glucocorticoids observed in all cells of our body. This noteworthy difference is attributable to the enhanced transport of amino acids into liver cells along with the increase in enzymes involved in protein synthesis in liver.

(c) *Increased transport of amino acids into hepatic cells and reduced transport of amino acids into extrahepatic cells.* The decreased transport of amino acids into extrahepatic cells decreases their intracellular amino acid concentrations and consequently decreases the synthesis of protein, while breakdown of proteins in the cells continues to release amino acids that diffuse out of the cells to increase the plasma amino acid concentration. Therefore, glucocorticoids mobilize amino acids from the extrahepatic tissues and thus diminish the tissue stores of protein. Subsequently, the increased plasma concentration of amino acids and their enhanced transport into the hepatic cells accounts for the following effects:

    1. Enhanced rate of deamination of amino acids by the liver
    2. Augmented protein synthesis in the liver
    3. Increased formation of plasma proteins by the liver
    4. Increased rate of gluconeogenesis (by conversion of amino acids to glucose).

**Fat Metabolism**

Glucocorticoids augment both the fatty acid mobilization and oxidation, but at the same time surplus levels are associated with a peculiar pattern of visceral obesity.

(a) *Mobilization of fatty acids.* Glucocorticoids promote mobilization of fatty acids from adipose tissue for gluconeogenesis. To some extent, this may be seen due to the reduced transport of glucose to the fat cells. For example, α-glycerophosphate (derived from glucose) is required for both deposition and maintenance of triglycerides in these cells. And in its absence, fat cells release fatty acids. Therefore, there is an increase in mobilization of fats along with enhanced oxidation of fatty acids that shift the metabolic pathways from utilization of glucose for energy to utilization of fatty acids in times of starvation or other stresses. This mechanism aids in long-term conservation of body glucose and glycogen by using fatty acids for metabolic energy.

(b) *Excess cortisol causes obesity.* Interestingly, despite its effect of increase in fatty acid mobilization and oxidation, excessive glucocorticoids cause a typical pattern of central obesity characterized by deposition of fat in the chest and head regions of the body, giving a buffalo-like torso and a rounded moon face. Although the underlying mechanism is still unclear, it has been speculated that the excess glucocorticoids also stimulate food intake, and also the rate of fat deposition at these sites is more than the rate of fat mobilization and oxidation. Also, glucocorticoids stimulate the adipocyte differentiation, promoting adipogenesis (through the transcriptional activation of key differentiation genes, including lipoprotein lipase, glycerol-3-phosphate dehydrogenase and leptin) more at these sites [17]. However, wasting of fat (and some supporting tissues) in the extremities produces thinning of the skin and fragility of cutaneous blood vessels typically seen in patients with excess glucocorticoids.

2. Bone and Calcium Metabolism

Excess glucocorticoids cause osteopenia and osteoporosis by inhibiting the function of bone-forming osteoblastic cells [18]. They may also cause osteonecrosis or avascular necrosis most frequently at the site of femur neck. They also induce negative calcium balance by inhibiting intestinal calcium absorption and increasing renal calcium excretion.

3. Salt and Water Homeostasis and Regulation of Blood Pressure

Glucocorticoids mediate their effects on salt and water balance primarily by acting on the kidney. They can possibly act on the mineralocorticoid receptors present on the distal nephron (depending on the activity of 11βHSD) to cause sodium and water retention and potassium loss [19]. However, at other sites of the nephron, glucocorticoids increase the glomerular filtration rate, proximal tubular epithelial sodium transport and free water clearance [20] and also reduce the levels of vasopressin. This final effect principally explains the phenomena of dilutional hyponatraemia observed in patients with glucocorticoid deficiency [21].

Glucocorticoids increase blood pressure by a dual mechanism by their action at the level of kidney and vasculature [22]. They have a permissive action for catecholamines and angiotensin II in vascular smooth muscle, wherein they increase the sensitivity for the action of these pressor hormones. At the same time, they supress the endothelial dilatation mediated by nitric oxide smooth muscle, and they increase the sensitivity to pressor agents such as catecholamines and angiotensin II while reducing nitric oxide-mediated endothelial dilatation. Glucocorticoids also increase the synthesis of angiotensinogen [23] and hence, acting via the renin-angiotensin-aldosterone axis, also affect the blood pressure. They can also result in the increase in myocardial contractility by augmenting the action of the catecholamines. Thus, glucocorticoids may be beneficial in shock to maintain the blood pressure.

4. Role in Stress

Stress is one of the most important stimuli for activation of hypothalamo-pituitary-adrenal (HPA) axis and causes an immediate and marked increase in ACTH secretion by the anterior pituitary gland, followed within minutes by greatly increased adrenocortical secretion of glucocorticoids. The significance of this rise in their levels in stressful situations is still not clear. One probable reason is that the glucocorticoids by their proteolytic and lipolytic actions cause rapid mobilization of amino acids and fats from cellular stores, thus making them immediately available both for energy and for synthesis of other compounds, including glucose, that may be needed by the body. Perhaps, it has been observed that sometimes the damaged tissues use the newly available amino acids to form new proteins that are essential to them. Also, these amino acids can possibly be utilized to synthesize other essential intracellular substances, such as purines, pyrimidines and creatine phosphate, which are imperative for maintenance of cellular life and reproduction. This speculation is supported by the fact that cortisol usually does not mobilize the basic functional proteins of the cells, such as the muscle contractile proteins and the proteins of neurons. This preferential effect of cortisol is beneficial in mobilizing only the labile proteins and therefore ensuring availability of amino acids to needy cells.

Apart from this glucocorticoids are required for the normal responses of vascular smooth muscle to the vasoconstrictor action of sympathetic nervous system in stress (permissive action of glucocorticoids).

5. Anti-inflammatory Actions and Effect on the Immune System

The normal response of the body to any tissue damage is inflammation. Although a protective response of our body, in some conditions, such as in rheumatoid arthritis, the inflammatory response goes overboard and is actually more damaging than the underlying disease itself. In these scenarios, it has been seen that administration of large amounts of cortisol not only ceases the inflammatory cascade but also reverses most of the already started effects of inflammation [24].

Before we understand the action of glucocorticoids, let us recapitulate the basic steps of inflammation as follows:

1. The first is the release of inflammatory mediators (such as histamine, bradykinin, proteolytic enzymes, prostaglandins and leukotrienes) from the damaged tissue cells.
2. This is followed by a stage of rubor or erythema characterized by an increase in blood flow to the inflamed area caused by the inflammatory mediators/chemokines released from the damaged tissues.
3. The next stage is oedema, which is the accumulation of plasma at the site of injury due to increased capillary permeability caused by chemokines. This may also be accompanied by clotting of the tissue fluid, resulting in non-pitting oedema.
4. Then there is migration of leukocytes at the site of damage again by chemoattractant effect of released inflammatory mediators.
5. After days or weeks, healing process is denoted by the process of fibrosis at the injured site.

Glucocorticoids halt this inflammatory process by two fundamental effects

1. It has the ability to block the early stages of the inflammatory process itself.
2. If inflammation has already started, it additionally has the potential to rapidly resolve and result in healing of the damaged tissue.

**Glucocorticoids Role in Blocking the Early Stages of Inflammation**
This effect is observed due to the following reasons (Fig. 5.5):

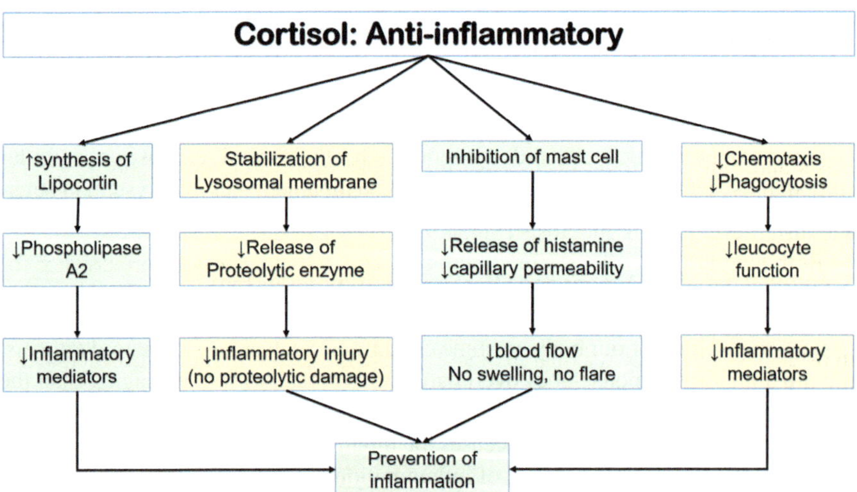


**Fig. 5.5** Anti-inflammatory action of glucocorticoids

1. Glucocorticoids stabilize the lysosomal membranes and thus prevent the release of the proteolytic enzymes that are released by damaged cells to cause inflammation
2. They also reduce the capillary permeability, probably by attenuating the effect of proteolytic enzymes and subsequently the manifestation of tissue oedema as well.
3. Moreover, they cause a reduction in migration of leukocytes to the inflamed area and also a decrease in phagocytosis of the damaged cells. This could be attributable to the diminish formation of chemokines like prostaglandins and leukotrienes that not only attenuate the vasodilation and capillary permeability but also reduce the chemo-attraction and mobility of white blood cells at the site of injury.
4. Additionally they suppress the production of lymphocyte, especially the T lymphocyte. This causes reduced inflammatory responses catered by the tissue reaction orchestrated by the T cells and antibodies.
5. Glucocorticoids also lessen the fever experienced during inflammation. This effect is due to its action of attenuating the release of interleukin1 from white blood cells which is responsible for mediating fever through its action on the hypothalamic temperature control system. This reduction in temperature subsequently not only reduces the degree of vasodilation but also hampers further tissue damage.

In this manner, glucocorticoids act in a holistic manner on almost all aspects of the inflammatory cascade and block its progression.

**Glucocorticoids' Role in Resolution of Already Ensued Inflammation**
Glucocorticoids are effective even after inflammation is established. They firstly attenuate all the factors (as discussed above) involved in inflammation and hence decrement the inflammatory response. Apart from this, they promote the rate of healing. Probable reasons for the above could be due to:

1. The proteolytic effect of glucocorticoids ensuring availability of amino acids for repair of the damaged tissues
2. The gluconeogenic effect of glucocorticoids that makes extra glucose available to the critical metabolic systems
3. The lipolytic effect and hence increased amounts of fatty acids are available for cellular energy.
4. Furthermore, it removes or inactivates certain inflammatory products.

The exact mechanism for the anti-inflammatory effect is still a matter of debate. But its major role in combating inflammation in many auto-immune diseases, like rheumatoid arthritis, rheumatic fever and acute glomerulonephritis to name a few, is proven beyond doubt. Moreover, even though the underlying disease pathology remains unaltered by glucocorticoids, they act lifesaving in these conditions by preventing the damaging effects of the inflammatory response itself.

**Glucocorticoids Also Attenuate the Inflammatory Response to Allergens**
Glucocorticoids are drug of choice in anaphylaxis and lifesaving as they prevent shock or death. Glucocorticoids help solely by blocking the inflammatory cascade (as discussed above).

**Glucocorticoids' Effect on Blood Cells and Immunity (Fig. 5.6)**
Glucocorticoids are known to decrease the number of basophils, eosinophils and lymphocytes in the blood by causing their redistribution from the intravascular compartment to the spleen, lymph nodes and bone marrow. Opposite to this, neutrophil counts increase after glucocorticoid administration. Also, administration of large doses of cortisol results in significant atrophy of lymphoid tissue throughout the body, thus reducing the production of T cells and antibodies from the lymphoid tissue. Additionally, glucocorticoids also inhibit the cytokine production from lymphocytes (by their anti-NF-κB action). NF-κB plays a significant role in inducing the cytokine gene transcription; glucocorticoids act in dual manner—firstly they bind directly to NF-κB and prevent its nuclear translocation, and secondly, they induce an NF-κB inhibitor, which sequesters NF-κB in the cytoplasm, thereby inactivating its effect [25]. Moreover, glucocorticoids also inhibit the inflammatory effects by inhibiting the differentiation of monocytes to macrophages and also reducing the phagocytic and cytotoxic potential of macrophages (in lieu of their lysosomal membrane stabilizing effects). They also reduce the secretion of the cytokine IL-2, thus diminishing the proliferation of lymphocytes and causing an increase in their apoptosis. As a consequence, the body's capability to mount an immune response to a foreign antigen reduces drastically. A noteworthy point is that glucocorticoids have little influence on the human immune system under normal physiologic conditions, and this immunosuppressive effect is observed only when large doses are administered over a prolonged period. This is the cause for avoiding

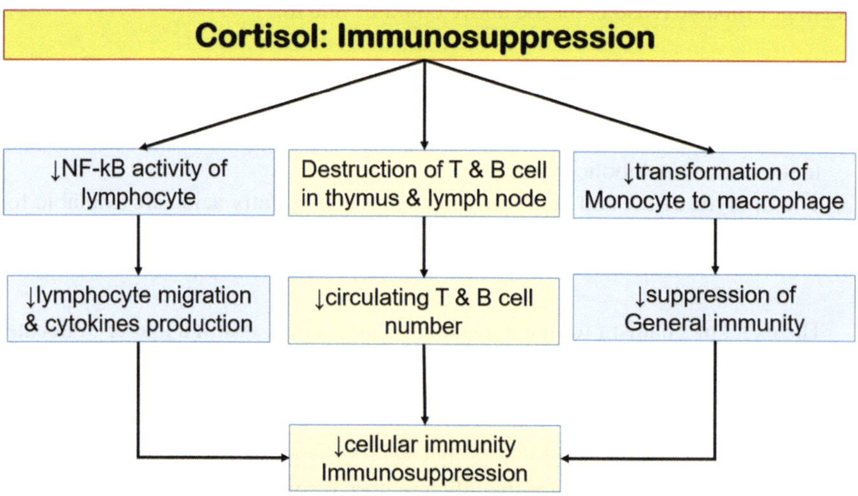


**Fig. 5.6** Immunosuppressive action of glucocorticoids

glucocorticoid administration in mild infection as the ensued immunosuppression could culminate to fulminating infection and death. While interestingly this same effect has been channelized to avoid immunological rejection of graft most commonly in kidney transplantation, glucocorticoids have also shown to increase the production of red blood cells and platelets by mechanisms that are unknown. Thus, in conditions with excess secretion of cortisol by the adrenal glands, polycythaemia is seen, and conversely, conditions with inadequate cortisol and anaemia are observed.

6. Permissive Action

Permissive action qualifies for those effects that are not primarily produced by glucocorticoids, but their presence (even though in minor amount) is required for that particular action. These include the requirement for glucocorticoids for the calorigenic effects of glucagon and catecholamines, for the lipolytic action of catecholamines and for the vascular reactivity and bronchodilatory effect of catecholamines.

7. Central Nervous System and Mood

Glucocorticoids affect the functioning of brain, and its defects are associated with a spectrum of manifestations ranging from depression, euphoria, psychosis, apathy and lethargy. Specifically, in adrenal insufficiency-irritability, apprehension and inability to concentrate and also electroencephalographic waves slower than normal β rhythm are observed. And all these are reversed by glucocorticoid therapy further emphasizing their effect on nervous system [2, 6].

8. Eye

Excess glucocorticoids have shown to raise the intraocular pressure by both—increasing the production of aqueous humour and preventing its drainage by enhancing deposition of matrix within the trabecular meshwork. This could attribute to the steroid-induced glaucoma observed in glucocorticoid excess [26].

9. Gut

Long-term administration of glucocorticoids has been associated with the risk of developing peptic ulcer disease [27]. Also, pancreatitis with fat necrosis has been observed in patients with glucocorticoid excess. Glucocorticoid receptors are expressed throughout the gastrointestinal tract, whereas mineralocorticoid receptor expression is highest in the distal colon; where they mediate the control of epithelial ion transport.

10. Growth and Development

In vitro glucocorticoids have shown to stimulate transcription of the gene encoding growth hormone (GH). However, conditions with glucocorticoid excess exhibit inhibition of linear skeletal growth [28, 29], probably due to the catabolic effects on connective tissue, muscle and bone and also through inhibition of the effects of insulin-like growth factor 1 (IGF1). Glucocorticoids also have an important role in the normal foetal development, most notably, in maturation of lungs through the synthesis of surfactant proteins (SP-A, SP-B and SP-C) [30]. They also stimulate the enzyme phenylethanolamine N-methyltransferase (PNMT), which converts noradrenaline to adrenaline in adrenal medulla and chromaffin tissue. Mice lacking the glucocorticoid receptor do not develop an adrenal medulla [31].

11. Endocrine Effects
Glucocorticoids suppress the secretion of thyroid-stimulating hormone (TSH). Moreover, they inhibit 5′ deiodinase enzyme activity that mediates the conversion of thyroxine to active triiodothyronine and thus hamper the thyroid hormone action.

They also act centrally to inhibit gonadotropin releasing hormone (GnRH) pulsatility and therefore the release of luteinizing hormone (LH) and follicle-stimulating hormone (FSH) and hence also affect the reproductive cycle.

#### 5.3.2.3 Adrenal Androgens

##### Biological Actions

Normally, the adrenal androgens have only weak effects in humans. It is postulated that part of the early development of the male sex organs is dependent on the childhood secretion of adrenal androgens. The adrenal androgens also exert minor effects in the female, not only before puberty but also throughout life. Much of the growth of the pubic and axillary hair in the female has been attributed to the action of these hormones. Excess adrenal androgens have a minimal effect in males, whose sexual characteristics are primarily affected by gonadal steroids (namely testosterone), while, in females, their excess can result in many androgen-like effects (like facial hair, etc.) and thus virilization. The major adrenal androgens are dehydroepiandrosterone (DHEA), androstenedione and 11-hydroxyandrostenedione. Both DHEA and androstenedione are weak androgens and are converted to testosterone in extraglandular tissues to mediate their androgenic effects. DHEA also has a few poorly understood effects on the immune and cardiovascular system. Adrenal androgen formation is regulated by ACTH and not by gonadotropins. Adrenal androgens are suppressed by exogenous glucocorticoid administration.

#### 5.3.2.4 Regulation of Adrenocortical Hormones

##### 1. Adrenocorticotropic Hormone

ACTH is the most important factor for regulation of the synthesis and secretion of glucocorticoids and androgens by the zona fasciculata and zona reticularis.

The factors that control ACTH release (Fig. 5.7) include hypothalamic corticotropin releasing hormone (CRH) [32], free plasma cortisol itself [33, 34] and the circadian rhythm [35]. Moreover, CRH release is caused by any stressful stimuli to the body (e.g., pyrogens, surgery, exercise, hypoglycaemia and severe emotional stimuli). Hypothalamic neurotransmitters modulate CRH release, serotoninergic and cholinergic systems stimulate the secretion of CRH and ACTH and adrenergic agonists and γ-aminobutyric acid (GABA) probably inhibit CRH release. Also,

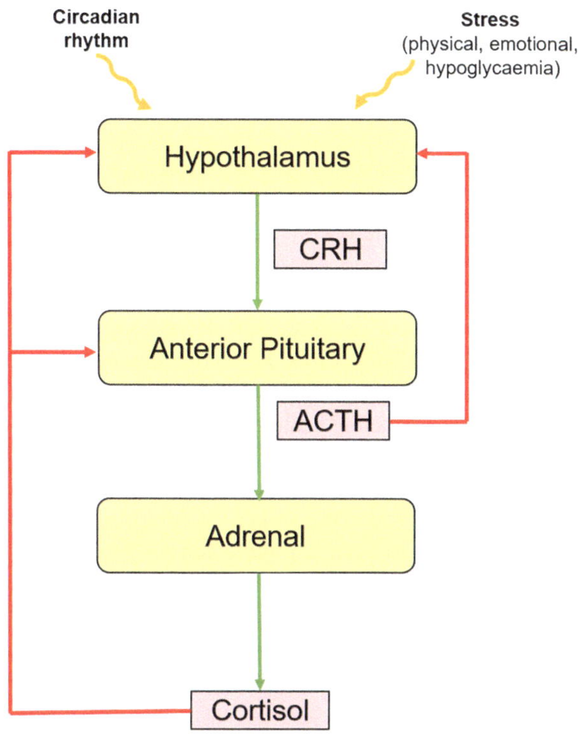


**Fig. 5.7** Hypothalamic-pituitary-adrenal axis. The hypothalamic CRH promotes the secretion of ACTH and some other peptides (namely MSH, β-LPT, etc.) from anterior pituitary which in turn stimulate the release of cortisol primarily from zona fasciculata. The main sites for negative feedback by free circulating cortisol are the pituitary gland itself and the hypothalamic corticotropin-releasing centre. Feedback control by plasma cortisol may also occur at the locus coeruleus/sympathetic system and some higher centres (not shown in figure) as well. There is also a short feedback loop involving inhibition of hypothalamic CRH by pituitary ACTH. *ACTH* adrenocorticotropic hormone, *β-LPT* β-lipotropin, *CRH* corticotropin-releasing hormone, *MSH* melanocyte-stimulating hormone

opioid peptides β-endorphin and enkephalin inhibit, while vasopressin and angiotensin II augment, the secretion of CRH and ACTH. The inflammatory cytokines [tumour necrosis factor-α (TNF-α) and interleukin (IL) 1α, IL-1β and IL-6] also stimulate CRH and/or vasopressin and hence enhance ACTH secretion [36].

The biologic half-life of ACTH in the circulation is less than 10 min. Additionally, the action of ACTH is also rapid; within minutes of its release, the level of cortisol in the adrenal venous blood rises. ACTH stimulates steroidogenesis via activation of adenylyl cyclase. Cyclic AMP, in turn, stimulates the synthesis of protein kinase enzymes, thereby resulting in the phosphorylation of proteins that activate the steroid biosynthesis process. Apart from it, it is also responsible for long-term trophic effects and maintains the cellular machinery necessary to carry out steroidogenesis at a rapid rate [37].

Another noteworthy point is the permissive role of ACTH for aldosterone secretion, wherein it is necessary but has little effect in controlling the rate of secretion in most physiological conditions.

**2. Angiotensin II**

The activation of renin-angiotensin system regulates extra-cellular fluid volume through aldosterone secretion. Angiotensin II stimulates the rate-limiting step in steroidogenesis to increase aldosterone synthesis [38].

**3. Potassium**

Potassium ion directly increases aldosterone synthesis and secretion by mediating transcriptional changes. Potassium depolarizes the membrane and increases intracellular calcium through opening of calcium channels which increase the activity of calmodulin kinases, independent of the circulating renin-angiotensin system, which it suppresses [38]. Additionally, it also has an indirect mechanism, where it modifies aldosterone secretion by activating the local renin-angiotensin system in the zona glomerulosa.

Moreover, having two different mechanisms of control— the HPA axis for glucocorticoid biosynthesis and the renin-angiotensin system for mineralocorticoid synthesis—has important clinical implications. Patients with primary adrenal failure have both cortisol and aldosterone deficiency, while patients with ACTH deficiency due to pituitary defect have only glucocorticoid deficiency but normal aldosterone concentrations because of the intact renin angiotensin system.

## 5.3.3 Applied Aspects

These could result from either a reduced secretion (hyposecretion) or increased secretion (hypersecretion). We will be discussing about them under these two subheadings.

### 5.3.3.1 Hyposecretion Disorders

**1. Adrenal Insufficiency**

Addison's disease (primary adrenal insufficiency) is characterized by insufficient adrenocortical hormones. This could be attributed due to either a primary atrophy or injury of the adrenal cortices. The most common cause of atrophy is autoimmune reaction. Additionally, it might also be observed due to tuberculous destruction of the adrenal glands or metastatic invasion of the adrenal cortices. Adrenal insufficiency may also be secondary to the impaired production of ACTH by the pituitary gland or tertiary due to inadequate CRH secretion by hypothalamus. Low ACTH levels not only reduce cortisol, adrenal androgens and to some extent aldosterone production but also lead to adrenal gland atrophy. Remarkably, secondary adrenal insufficiency is much more common than Addison's disease. Also, both secondary and tertiary are usually milder than primary adrenal insufficiency as electrolyte homeostasis is less affected in them. Another noteworthy difference between them is the plasma levels of ACTH which are low in secondary and tertiary and high in primary adrenal insufficiency. Additionally, isolated aldosterone deficiency has also been reported in patients with renal disease and also a low circulating renin level (hyporeninemic hypoaldosteronism). Apart from this, there is also a disorder named as pseudo-hypoaldosteronism which is most commonly due to an aldosterone receptor defect resulting in resistance to the action of aldosterone. Adrenal insufficiency will have manifestations due to decrease in all the hormones secreted by the adrenal cortices, while those with only aldosterone defects have symptoms limited to deficiency of mineralocorticoids [39].

**Manifestations Due to Mineralocorticoid Deficiency**

Lack of mineralocorticoid secretion causes a marked decrease in extracellular fluid volume by decreasing the renal tubular sodium reabsorption and consequently allowing great loss of sodium ions, chloride ions and water in urine. Moreover, along with hyponatraemia and hyperkalaemia, mild acidosis also develops because of failure of potassium and hydrogen ions to be secreted in exchange for sodium reabsorption. As the extracellular fluid becomes depleted, plasma volume also falls, and red blood cell concentration rises markedly, cardiac output and blood pressure decrease and the patient may die in shock.

**Manifestations Due to Glucocorticoid Deficiency**

Loss of glucocorticoid secretion majorly affects the blood glucose concentration between meals because the patient is unable to synthesize significant quantities of glucose by gluconeogenesis. Also, there is reduced mobilization of both proteins and fats from the tissues, thereby perturbing many other metabolic functions of the body. This hampering of energy mobilization is one of the most detrimental effects of glucocorticoid deficiency. Moreover, even when excess quantities of glucose and other nutrients are available, patients with Addison's disease have weak muscles, further emphasizing that glucocorticoids are essential to maintain other metabolic functions of the tissues in addition to energy metabolism. These patients are more prone to the deteriorating effects of any type stress, and thus even a mild respiratory infection can cause death in them.

**Manifestations of Adrenal Androgens Deficiency**

Mild menstrual abnormalities might occur in women, but mostly the deficiency of adrenal androgens usually has little effect in the presence of normal testes or ovaries.

**Melanin Pigmentation**

Another typical feature of most people with Addison's disease is melanin pigmentation of the mucous membranes and skin. The underlying mechanism of the excessive melanin deposition is speculated to be due to the simultaneous increase in MSH and ACTH secretion. The decrease in glucocorticoids causes less negative feedback to the hypothalamus and anterior pituitary gland, therefore resulting in tremendous rise in ACTH secretion along with MSH. The large amounts of ACTH may also stimulate formation of melanin by the melanocytes in the same way that MSH does [39, 40].

**Addisonian Crisis**

This a term used for a special situation in patients of Addison's disease—wherein the body critically requires extra glucocorticoids and suffers severe debility in its absence, especially in state of any stress. As discussed earlier in this chapter, an increase in glucocorticoids secretions is necessarily required for body's response to different types of physical or mental stress. In Addison's disease, the output of glucocorticoids does not increase as per the requirements during stress, and consequently the patients have major incapacity to handle stress.

### 5.3.3.2 Hypersecretion Disorders

#### 1. Cushing's Syndrome

Hypersecretion by the adrenal cortex causes Cushing's syndrome—a disease characterized by a multitude of characteristic clinical features due to hormone excess. Most of the abnormal manifestations of Cushing's syndrome are attributable to excessive glucocorticoids, but enhanced secretion of androgens may also result in some important effects [41].

Multiple aetiologies could result in Cushing's syndrome, including:

1. Adenomas of the anterior pituitary that secrete large amounts of ACTH, which then causes adrenal hyperplasia and excess glucocorticoid secretion (also referred to as Cushing's disease)
2. Abnormality at the level of hypothalamus that causes secretion of excess corticotropin releasing hormone, which in turn stimulates the excess ACTH release from pituitary and consequently more glucocorticoid secretion
3. 'Ectopic secretion' of ACTH by a tumour elsewhere in the body, such as an abdominal carcinoma
4. Adenomas of the adrenal cortex

Cushing's syndrome due to excess ACTH secretion is more common and is characterized by high plasma levels of both ACTH and cortisol (the most abundant glucocorticoid), while primary overproduction of cortisol by the adrenal glands accounts only for about 20 to 25 percent of clinical cases of Cushing's syndrome and is usually associated with reduced ACTH levels and high cortisol due to the excessive feedback inhibition of ACTH secretion by the anterior pituitary gland. Administration of large doses of dexamethasone, a synthetic glucocorticoid, can be used to distinguish between ACTHdependent and ACTHindependent Cushing's syndrome. In patients with overproduction of ACTH due to an ACTH-secreting pituitary adenoma or to hypothalamic-pituitary dysfunction, low doses of dexamethasone fail to suppress ACTH secretion normally. However, by increasing the dose of dexamethasone to very high levels, ACTH eventually can be suppressed in most patients with Cushing's disease (ACTH-dependent). In contrast, patients with primary adrenal overproduction of glucocorticoids (ACTH-independent Cushing's syndrome) usually have low or undetectable levels of ACTH. The limitation of this dexamethasone suppression is that some ACTH-secreting pituitary tumours variants do respond to low dose dexamethasone with suppressed ACTH secretion.

Additionally, nonpituitary ectopic malignant tumours that produce ACTH, such as certain lung carcinomas, are not responsive to the glucocorticoid-negative feedback. Still, the dexamethasone test is usually considered to be a first step in the differential diagnosis of Cushing's syndrome. Cushing's syndrome may also be iatrogenically induced due to over enthusiastic administration of large amounts of glucocorticoids over prolonged periods for therapeutic purposes. For example, patients with rheumatoid arthritis are often treated with glucocorticoids to deal with the chronic inflammation in this disorder, and consequently these patients may experience some of the clinical symptoms of Cushing's syndrome due to glucocorticoid excess.

**Clinical Features (Fig. 5.8) [41–44]**

1. Central obesity

There is mobilization of fat from the lower part of the body, with concomitant extra deposition of fat in the thoracic and upper abdominal regions, giving rise to a

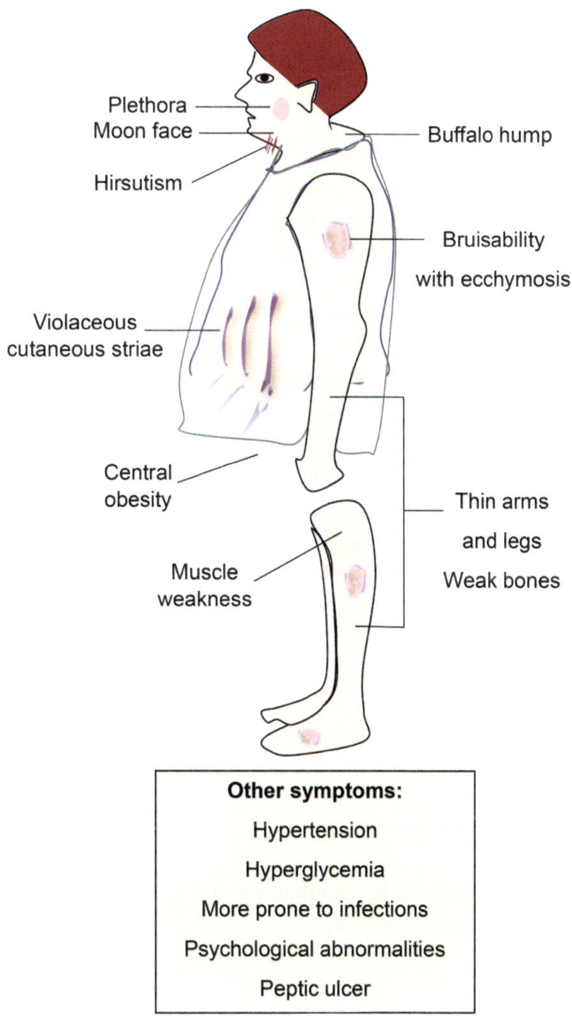


**Fig. 5.8** Classical clinical features of Cushing's syndrome

buffalo-like torso. Similarly, excessive deposition of facial fat and oedema gives a characteristic moon face appearance.

2. Acne and hirsutism

There is also associated excess secretion of androgens that may cause acne and hirsutism (excess growth of facial hair) and also amenorrhoea.

3. Hypertension

Around 80 percent of patients also have hypertension, probably due to effects of excess glucocorticoids on the mineralocorticoid receptor and hence sodium and water retention.

4. Hyperglycaemia

There is an increase in blood glucose concentration due to the effects of glucocorticoids on carbohydrate metabolism, mainly due to enhanced gluconeogenesis and decreased glucose utilization by the tissues.

5. Muscle weakness

The excess glucocorticoids result in protein catabolism throughout the body (with the exception of the liver). This extreme loss of protein especially from the muscles causes severe weakness.

6. More prone to infections

The associated loss of protein synthesis in the lymphoid tissues culminates to a suppressed immune system, and thus patients fail to deal with infections.

7. Violaceous striae and ecchymosis

Subcutaneous tissue tears easily due to loss of the protein collagen fibres and results in easy bruisability and subsequently development of large violaceous purplish striae.

8. Osteoporosis

Also, a decrease in protein deposition in the bones often causes severe osteoporosis with consequent weakness of the bones.

9. Plethoric appearance

Glucocorticoids stimulate the red cell production and thus may result in a characteristic facial plethora.

10. Mental abnormalities

A whole range of psychiatric abnormalities are observable ranging from insomnia, depression to psychosis attributable to the effect of excess glucocorticoids on central nervous system.

**2. Hyperaldosteronism**

Hypersecretion of aldosterone by a tumour of the zona glomerulosa cells itself (due to either an adenoma or adrenal carcinoma or unilateral or bilateral adrenal hyperplasia) is called as primary aldosteronism or Conn's syndrome, while secondary hyperaldosteronism is caused by liver cirrhosis, heart failure and nephrosis. The most important effects of hyperaldosteronism are hypokalaemia, mild metabolic alkalosis, a slight increase in extracellular fluid volume and blood volume, a modest increase in plasma sodium concentration (usually <4–6 mEq/L increase) and hypertension. Especially a noteworthy manifestation in primary aldosteronism patients is the occasional periods of muscle paralysis caused by the hypokalaemia. Hypokalaemia causes decrement in the action potential transmission by the nerve fibres and concomitant paralysis. The decrease in plasma renin concentration is one of the diagnostic criteria of primary aldosteronism. This characteristic decrease in renin is due to two main reasons:

- Excess aldosterone due to feedback inhibition results in decrease in renin levels.
- The excess extracellular fluid volume and arterial pressure (consequent to high circulating aldosterone) cause decrease in stimuli for renin secretion.

However, secondary hyperaldosteronism is associated with a high plasma renin activity.

Also, usually there is slight sodium and fluid retention but without oedema. These patients can also manifest hypocalcaemic tetany due to the accompanying metabolic alkalosis [9, 45].

**3. Adrenogenital Syndrome**

This is caused by an occasional adrenocortical tumour secreting excess quantities of androgens. These androgens further cause intense masculinizing effects throughout the body. In women with adrenogenital syndrome, virile characteristics are quite appreciable, including the growth of a beard, a deeper voice, male pattern baldness, masculine distribution of hair on the body and the pubis, growth of the clitoris to resemble a penis and deposition of proteins in the skin and especially in the muscles to give typical masculine characteristics and can sometimes also cause female pseudo-hermaphroditism. In the prepubertal male, a virilizing adrenal tumour causes the same characteristics as in the female along with a rapid development of the male sexual organs resulting in precocious pseudo-puberty. However, in an adult male, the virilizing characteristics of adrenogenital syndrome are usually obscured by the normal virilizing characteristics of the testosterone (the major androgen) secreted by the testes. It is often difficult to make a diagnosis of adrenogenital syndrome in the adult male based on the clinical features, while biochemically the excretion of 17-ketosteroids (which are derived from androgens) in the urine may be 10–15 times normal, and this can be utilized in diagnosing the disease.

## 5.4 Other Applied Aspects

### 5.4.1 Medical Use of Glucocorticoids

Glucocorticoids have been effectively utilized in several medical conditions as listed below:

- As replacement therapy for patients suffering from either adrenal insufficiency or congenital enzyme disorders resulting in congenital adrenal hyperplasia (CAH)
- As treatment of various forms of allergic responses
- Renal disease (nephrotic syndrome)
- Asthma
- Autoimmune disease
- Also, for immunosuppression in various organ transplants, most commonly renal transplant

## References

1. Gwynne JT, Strauss JF. The role of lipoproteins in steroidogenesis and cholesterol metabolism in steroidogenic glands. Endocr Rev. 1982;3(3):299–329.
2. Williams textbook of endocrinology—13th Edition [Internet]. [cited 2020 Jul 2]. Available from: https://www.elsevier.com/books/williams-textbook-of-endocrinology/9780323297387
3. Speiser PW, White PC. Congenital adrenal hyperplasia. N Engl J Med. 2003;349(8):776–88.
4. Buy medical physiology (medical physiology (Rhoades)) book online at low prices in India | medical physiology (medical physiology (Rhoades)) reviews & ratings—Amazon.in [Internet]. [cited 2020 Jul 2]. Available from: https://www.amazon.in/Medical-Physiology-Rhoades/dp/0781719364
5. Chapman K, Holmes M, Seckl J. 11β-hydroxysteroid dehydrogenases: intracellular gate-keepers of tissue glucocorticoid action. Physiol Rev. 2013;93(3):1139–206.
6. Buy Ganong's review of medical physiology, twenty-fifth edition (Lange medical book) book online at low prices in India | Ganong's review of medical physiology, twenty-fifth edition (Lange medical book) reviews & ratings—Amazon.in [Internet]. [cited 2020 Jul 2]. Available from: https://www.amazon.in/Ganongs-Review-Medical-Physiology-Twenty-Fifth/dp/007182510X
7. Hammond GL. Molecular properties of corticosteroid binding globulin and the sex-steroid binding proteins. Endocr Rev. 1990;11(1):65–79.
8. Fukushima DK, Bradlow HL, Hellman L, Zumoff B, Gallagher TF. Metabolic transformation of hydrocortisone-4-C14 in normal men. J Biol Chem. 1960;235:2246–52.
9. Fuller PJ. Adrenal diagnostics: an endocrinologist's perspective focused on hyperaldosteronism. Clin Biochem Rev. 2013;34(3):111–6.

10. Funder JW. Minireview: aldosterone and the cardiovascular system: genomic and nongenomic effects. Endocrinology. 2006;147(12):5564–7.
11. Guichard JL, Clark D, Calhoun DA, Ahmed MI. Aldosterone receptor antagonists: current perspectives and therapies. Vasc Health Risk Manag. 2013;9:321–31.
12. Buy Harrison's endocrinology, 4E (Harrison's specialty) book online at low prices in India | Harrison's endocrinology, 4E (Harrison's specialty) reviews & ratings—Amazon.in [Internet]. [cited 2020 Jul 2]. Available from: https://www.amazon.in/Harrisons-Endocrinology-4E-Specialty/dp/1259835723
13. Pratt WB. The role of heat shock proteins in regulating the function, folding, and trafficking of the glucocorticoid receptor. J Biol Chem. 1993;268(29):21455–8.
14. Beato M, Sánchez-Pacheco A. Interaction of steroid hormone receptors with the transcription initiation complex. Endocr Rev. 1996;17(6):587–609.
15. Chakravarty K, Cassuto H, Reshef L, Hanson RW. Factors that control the tissue-specific transcription of the gene for phosphoenolpyruvate carboxykinase-C. Crit Rev Biochem Mol Biol. 2005;40(3):129–54.
16. Olefsky JM. Effect of dexamethasone on insulin binding, glucose transport, and glucose oxidation of isolated rat adipocytes. J Clin Invest. 1975;56(6):1499–508.
17. Hauner H, Entenmann G, Wabitsch M, Gaillard D, Ailhaud G, Negrel R, et al. Promoting effect of glucocorticoids on the differentiation of human adipocyte precursor cells cultured in a chemically defined medium. J Clin Invest. 1989;84(5):1663–70.
18. Canalis E. Clinical review 83: mechanisms of glucocorticoid action in bone: implications to glucocorticoid-induced osteoporosis. J Clin Endocrinol Metab. 1996;81(10):3441–7.
19. Quinkler M, Stewart PM. Hypertension and the cortisol-cortisone shuttle. J Clin Endocrinol Metab. 2003;88(6):2384–92.
20. Marver D. Evidence of corticosteroid action along the nephron. Am J Physiol. 1984;246(2 Pt 2):F111–23.
21. Raff H. Glucocorticoid inhibition of neurohypophysial vasopressin secretion. Am J Physiol. 1987;252(4 Pt 2):R635–44.
22. Fraser R, Davies DL, Connell JM. Hormones and hypertension. Clin Endocrinol (Oxf). 1989;31(6):701–46.
23. Saruta T, Suzuki H, Handa M, Igarashi Y, Kondo K, Senba S. Multiple factors contribute to the pathogenesis of hypertension in Cushing's syndrome. J Clin Endocrinol Metab. 1986;62(2):275–9.
24. Petta I, Dejager L, Ballegeer M, Lievens S, Tavernier J, De Bosscher K, et al. The interactome of the glucocorticoid receptor and its influence on the actions of glucocorticoids in combatting inflammatory and infectious diseases. Microbiol Mol Biol Rev MMBR. 2016;80(2):495–522.
25. McKay LI, Cidlowski JA. Molecular control of immune/inflammatory responses: interactions between nuclear factor-kappa B and steroid receptor-signaling pathways. Endocr Rev. 1999;20(4):435–59.
26. Clark AF. Basic sciences in clinical glaucoma: steroids, ocular hypertension, and glaucoma. J Glaucoma. 1995;4(5):354–69.
27. Messer J, Reitman D, Sacks HS, Smith H, Chalmers TC. Association of adrenocorticosteroid therapy and peptic-ulcer disease. N Engl J Med. 1983;309(1):21–4.
28. Strickland AL, Underwood LE, Voina SJ, French FS, Van Wyk JJ. Growth retardation in Cushing's syndrome. Am J Dis Child 1960. 1972;123(3):207–213.
29. Leonard MB, Feldman HI, Shults J, Zemel BS, Foster BJ, Stallings VA. Long-term, high-dose glucocorticoids and bone mineral content in childhood glucocorticoid-sensitive nephrotic syndrome. N Engl J Med. 2004;351(9):868–75.
30. Ballard PL, Ertsey R, Gonzales LW, Gonzales J. Transcriptional regulation of human pulmonary surfactant proteins SP-B and SP-C by glucocorticoids. Am J Respir Cell Mol Biol. 1996;14(6):599–607.
31. Cole TJ, Blendy JA, Monaghan AP, Krieglstein K, Schmid W, Aguzzi A, et al. Targeted disruption of the glucocorticoid receptor gene blocks adrenergic chromaffin cell development and severely retards lung maturation. Genes Dev. 1995;9(13):1608–21.

32. Rivier C, Rivier J, Vale W. Inhibition of adrenocorticotropic hormone secretion in the rat by immunoneutralization of corticotropin-releasing factor. Science. 1982;218(4570):377–9.
33. Lundblad JR, Roberts JL. Regulation of proopiomelanocortin gene expression in pituitary. Endocr Rev. 1988;9(1):135–58.
34. Keller-Wood ME, Dallman MF. Corticosteroid inhibition of ACTH secretion. Endocr Rev. 1984;5(1):1–24.
35. Weitzman ED, Fukushima D, Nogeire C, Roffwarg H, Gallagher TF, Hellman L. Twenty-four hour pattern of the episodic secretion of cortisol in normal subjects. J Clin Endocrinol Metab. 1971;33(1):14–22.
36. Bateman A, Singh A, Kral T, Solomon S. The immune-hypothalamic-pituitary-adrenal axis. Endocr Rev. 1989;10(1):92–112.
37. Simpson ER, Waterman MR. Regulation of the synthesis of steroidogenic enzymes in adrenal cortical cells by ACTH. Annu Rev Physiol. 1988;50:427–40.
38. Rainey WE. Adrenal zonation: clues from 11beta-hydroxylase and aldosterone synthase. Mol Cell Endocrinol. 1999;151(1–2):151–60.
39. Charmandari E, Nicolaides NC, Chrousos GP. Adrenal insufficiency. Lancet Lond Engl. 2014;383(9935):2152–67.
40. Bornstein SR. Predisposing factors for adrenal insufficiency. N Engl J Med. 2009;360(22):2328–39.
41. Prague JK, May S, Whitelaw BC. Cushing's syndrome. BMJ. 2013;346:f945.
42. Findling JW, Raff H. Cushing's syndrome: important issues in diagnosis and management. J Clin Endocrinol Metab. 2006;91(10):3746–53.
43. Tritos NA, Biller BMK. Advances in medical therapies for Cushing's syndrome. Discov Med. 2012;13(69):171–9.
44. Boscaro M, Arnaldi G. Approach to the patient with possible Cushing's syndrome. J Clin Endocrinol Metab. 2009;94(9):3121–31.
45. Gomez-Sanchez CE, Oki K. Minireview: potassium channels and aldosterone dysregulation: is primary aldosteronism a potassium channelopathy? Endocrinology. 2014;155(1):47–55.

# Pineal Gland and Circadian Rhythms: Melatonin and Sleep–Wake Cycle Regulation

6

Tania Talwar

**Abstract**

The pineal gland acts like a bridge between the nervous and endocrine systems, to serve as the principle regulator of circadian rhythms. The history of pineal research starting with philosophical speculation to its current emergence as a neuroendocrine organ is discussed in this chapter. The chapter also provides an overview of circadian rhythms, their fundamental properties, organization, and the role of the suprachiasmatic nucleus as the master pacemaker. A special emphasis has been made on the genetic and molecular mechanisms underlying circadian oscillations, including core clock genes and transcription–translation feedback loops. Pineal gland anatomy, development, functions, and mechanism of action of its principle hormone have also been discussed. The discovery, biosynthesis, regulation, secretion, and metabolism of melatonin, along with its physiological actions on various systems, are described. Emerging evidence linking circadian disruption and melatonin signaling to metabolic disorders and cancer biology is also discussed. This chapter underscores the pineal gland's essential role in maintaining temporal homeostasis and coordinating systemic physiology with environmental light–dark cycles.

**Keywords**

Pineal gland · Melatonin · Circadian rhythms · Suprachiasmatic nucleus · Sleep–wake cycle · Light–dark cycle · Chronobiology · Biological clock · Clock genes · Transcription–translation feedback loop · Neuroendocrine regulation

T. Talwar (✉)
Department of Physiology, All India Institute of Medical Sciences, New Delhi, India





H. Prabhakar, M. Kaur (eds.), *Brain and Endocrine Crosstalk*, Physiology in Clinical Neurosciences – Brain and Spinal Cord Crosstalks,
https://doi.org/10.1007/978-981-92-0763-3_6

## 6.1 Introduction

Although the pineal gland has been well known for more than 2000 years, the history of pineal research is full of alternating periods of stagnation and progress. Kappers [1], in his survey *Short History of Pineal Discovery and Research*, divided the history of pineal gland into three periods. The first period in the history of pineal research spans from around 300 B.C. to the mid-nineteenth century and is marked largely by speculation influenced by dominant philosophical ideologies and limited scientific knowledge. Research during this era was hindered by a lack of empirical methods and inadequate investigative tools. The pineal gland was likely first identified in humans by Herophilos (325–280 B.C.), an anatomist at the University of Alexandria, whose original works have been lost but were later cited by Galen (130–300 A.D.). Herophilos is also thought to have been among the first to associate the soul with the brain's ventricular system. He viewed the pineal gland as a kind of tap controlling the flow of "pneuma" (or "spiritus" in Latin) between the third and fourth ventricles. At the time, it was believed that air inhaled into the lungs traveled to the heart, where it became "*pneuma zotikon*" (vital spirit), which then transformed into "*pneuma psychikon*" (animal spirit) in the brain. This latter form of spirit, influenced by sensory perception, was thought to be responsible for the formation of knowledge. Although Galen accepted the concept of the *pneuma*, he rejected the idea that the pineal gland functioned as a tap for the brain's ventricular system, rightly noting that it lay outside this system. He named the pineal body "*soma konoeides*" or *konareion*, Latin for *conarium*, because of its close resemblance to a pine cone. Andreas Vesalius (1514–1564), in his seminal work *De Humani Corporis Fabrica Libri Septem* (1543), provided one of the earliest anatomical descriptions of the pineal gland. He discussed the structure and consistency of the gland but had no mention about its possible function. Like Galen, Vesalius also rejected the idea that the gland could be responsible for controlling the flow between the third and fourth ventricles. A few years later, René Descartes (1596–1650), known for claiming the pineal gland as the "seat of the soul," brought a new philosophical description about the pineal structure. Descartes' views came at a time when the question of the exact location of the "soul" of the human body was a concern among both philosophers and scientists alike. Descartes emphasized that the soul, in essence, cannot be thought of as confined or limited to a specific organ of the body. He proposed that the most direct expression of the soul was through the pineal gland, the only unpaired part of the brain. According to him, the pineal gland was responsible for production of the "*esprits animaux*," a refined substance derived from the finest particles of the blood. This suggestion echoed that of *spiritus animalis* of earlier classical thinkers. According to them, the animal spirits were thought to flow into minute openings or "*poroi*" that were present along the walls of the ventricles of brain. These pores acted as points of entry into small tubular nerves that originated from the ventricular surfaces. According to Descartes' model, sensory impressions like images formed on the retina would pass through the optic nerves, via hollow tubes, finally entering into the ventricular system. From the ventricles, these impressions of these images travel through the pores or openings into the pineal gland or "gland H." The pineal or "gland H" would then give out motor responses to the impressions of these images by sending animal spirits into the corresponding motor nerves. The gland could channel spirits into different pores simply by shifting its position in turn activating various motor pathways. Apart from this mechanical explanation, Descartes also proposed that there was an *âme raisonnable* or a rational soul, which influenced the activity of the pineal gland. The existence of two distinct types of principles, separating the mind which was responsible for thinking and the body as its physical extension, formed the core of Descartes' philosophy.

The second period from mid-nineteenth century till about the mid-twentieth century saw a revival of interest in the pineal organ. This interest was mainly in the field of pineal comparative anatomy, histology, and embryology. In terms of comparative anatomy, Ahlborn (1884) and Rabl-Riickhardt (1886) pointed out the analogy between the vesicular nonmammalian pineal organ and the primary optic vesicles. Studnicka stated that many of the characteristics of the mammalian pineal organ would point to a glandular function, by drawing comparison to the rudimental vestige of the well-developed nonmammalian organ. In the mammalian pineal organ, Studnicka distinguished typical cells, later identified as pinealocytes, and neuroglial cells. The presence of granules and vesicles in the first cell type was suggestive of their secretory activity. Hence by the mid-twentieth century, the main line along which the phylogenetic evolution of the pineal organ proceeded was established.

A sharp boundary between the second and the third period of pineal research cannot easily be drawn. However, during this period, knowledge of pineal physiology and endocrinology was decisively shaped by two seminal contributions. The first in 1954 by Kitay and Altschule, in their work *The Pineal Gland*, provided the first comprehensive synthesis of knowledge on the organ. Subsequently in 1958, Lerner's isolation and structural characterization of melatonin catalyzed extensive investigations by biochemists, anatomists, and physiologists into pineal structure and function. This body of work was then unified by Wurtman and Axelrod in 1965, establishing the concept of the pineal organ as a neuroendocrine sensor and actuator.

Figure 6.1 outlines the various neural, neurohormonal, hormonal, and neurohumoral inputs, and the various outputs of the mammalian pineal gland are shown, highlighting its role in locomotion, sleep, and endocrine control.

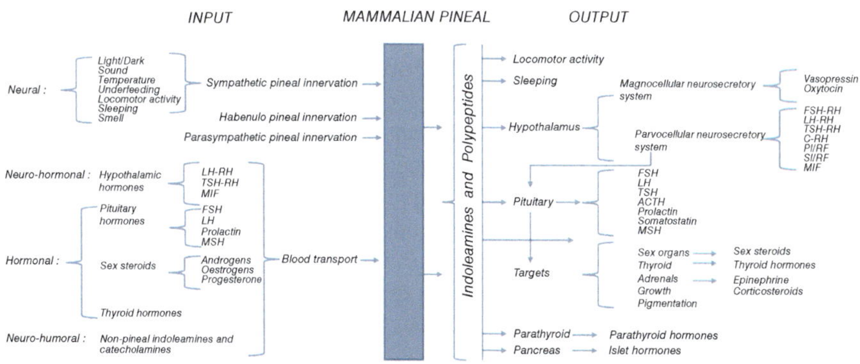


**Fig. 6.1** The inputs to pineal are represented on the left panel. On the right, the various outputs of the mammalian pineal gland are shown. The feedback mechanisms and several hormones regulated by pineal and their reciprocal influence on pineal activity have also been mentioned [1]

## 6.2 Circadian Rhythms and Sleep–Wake Cycle

The rotation of the Earth on its axis, occurring approximately every 24 h, results in environmental alternating fluctuations in light and temperature. This creates a time-based daily rhythmic pattern. All organisms on Earth are subjected to these daily patterns of fluctuations. In order to anticipate and adapt to these daily oscillations, these organisms, from the smallest cyanobacteria to humans, have evolved internal clocks. Several physiological processes have accordingly been synchronized with this internal clock or time-based system [2].

The earliest documented evidence linking physiology and the Earth's rotation resulting in a repetitive time-based changes in light dates back to the year 1729, when observations of the plant *Mimosa pudica* revealed that the leaves of *mimosa* opened during the day and closed in the night. This rhythmic pattern of opening and closing of leaves persisted even when there was continuous darkness, and the plant was deprived of all temporal indices and external light cues [3]. This persistent rhythmic biological pattern even under experimental conditions indicated that there existed an endogenous timing mechanism within the plant. It is now well established that the biological rhythms and patterns are intrinsic or in-built. The periodic cycles of organism physiology and behavior such as sleep–wake patterns, fluctuations in body temperature, and hormone secretion are all driven by internal clocks. Early research in the field of biological rhythms focused on cycles with a 24-h period, known as circadian rhythms (circa means about, and diem means day). The circadian rhythms with a ~24-h periodicity were not only perfectly aligned with the light–dark cycle but also known to persist without external cues. Ultradian rhythms (with a duration of less than 90 min) and infradian rhythms (with a duration of more than 28 h) complemented circadian oscillations. The three types of rhythms together formed an integrated temporal network which was essential for physiological regulation. Any disruption in these rhythms made the body vulnerable to psychological, metabolic, and cardiovascular disorders and impaired sleep, attention, and vigilance.

### 6.2.1 Chronobiology: Characteristics and Fundamental Principles of Circadian Rhythms

Since the observation in 1729 in *mimosa* plant that circadian rhythms persisted even in the absence of external cues, the fundamental principles that define modern circadian chronobiology have been worked upon by temporal isolation studies. All of these studies concluded that circadian rhythms follow and match with the 24-h solar day. The rhythms undergo only minimal variations (approximately 0.55% in humans) due to strict genetic regulation of the endogenous clock. The studies also inferred that in the absence of external cues, circadian rhythms persisted as self-sustained periodic patterns of oscillation, also due to the existence of the internal timekeeping system. In the studies, circadian rhythms were shown to be susceptible to alterations by extraneous changes (e.g., photoentrainment), and their periodicity remained consistent across wide temperature variations (temperature compensation).

The studies also provide evidence indicating toward a cell-driven genetic mechanism that underlies the human circadian clock and generates intrinsic rhythmicity. Under normal conditions, circadian rhythms are synchronized by environmental stimuli. Such external environmental cues, termed *zeitgebers* (German for "time givers"), have the capability to entrain human circadian rhythms.

The sleep–wake cycle that was once thought to operate with a periodicity of ~25 h lead to confounding of accurate circadian assessment. This was because the sleep–wake cycle was characterized under experimental light conditions that resulted in inaccurate assessment. Subsequent healthy human studies relied on the use of precise physiological markers such as melatonin levels, fluctuations in the core body temperature, and cortisol secretion, in addition to the light conditions. These studies helped demonstrate that the intrinsic human circadian pacemaker averages 24.18 h, under strict controlled light conditions. This value was also comparable to that observed in other species. The conclusion of all these experiments was that light serves as the primary *zeitgeber* across all species and was capable of producing phase shifts. These extent and direction of these shifts depended on the phase of exposure to light. It is now well established that daily rhythms arise from endogenous oscillators and that photosensitive organisms, subjected to recurring environmental cycles, have evolved behavioral, physiological, and metabolic rhythms aligned to the ~24 h circadian cycle.

### 6.2.2 Parameters of Circadian Rhythms

Circadian rhythms operate at multiple levels, from intracellular processes, such as gene expression, cell signaling, and proliferation, to tissue, organ, and systemic functions. These rhythms are characterized by specific parameters:

- Period (the duration of one oscillatory cycle)
- Amplitude (the intensity of rhythmic variation, typically measured as the difference between peak and midpoint or half of peak-to-trough value)
- Phase (the position of a cycle relative to a reference point, such as night onset)

While circadian rhythms persist and operate even without extraneous cues, their presence usually leads the rhythms to align accordingly. Entrainment, such as during transmeridian travel, can lead to shift in the position of the cycle forward or backward, resulting in their advancement or delay in the phase. In humans, these processes are controlled and coordinated by a circadian timing system or the master biological clock.

## 6.3 Suprachiasmatic Nucleus: The Body's Master Clock

The master pacemaker of the clock is the suprachiasmatic nuclei (SCN), located bilaterally in the anterior hypothalamus. This master clock serves as the central circadian regulator and pacemaker in a hierarchically organized system. It helps in coordinating the peripheral oscillators through neural and neuroendocrine pathways. The SCN regulates almost all mammalian circadian rhythms. In vivo and in vitro studies reveal that the SCN is a heterogeneous neuronal network which is capable of sustaining rhythmic activity and hence is called the master pacemaker. Lesion-based experiments demonstrate that SCN ablation abolishes behavioral rhythmicity, whereas SCN transplants restore rhythms in most arrhythmic hosts, with the restored period matching the donor genotype. Beyond free-running rhythmicity, the SCN enables organisms to anticipate and synchronize with environmental cycles, thereby maintaining temporal organization and homeostasis. At the cellular level, circadian timing arises from self-sustained molecular feedback loops with ~24-h periodicity, driven by clock genes expressed in the SCN and in peripheral tissues and organs.

### 6.3.1 Genetic Basis of the Biological Clock and Rhythms

The SCN comprises individual cellular circadian oscillators. They are well coordinated and operate in unison to generate observable rhythms via integrated outputs. In mammals, nearly all ~20,000 SCN neurons are believed to function as clock cells. Approximately 50% of the protein-coding genes exhibit circadian transcription in at least one human tissue, regulated by intrinsic transcription–translation feedback loops (TTFLs) [4–30]. At the cellular level, circadian oscillations arise from the rhythmic expression of core clock genes and their protein products. The molecular machinery of the circadian clock is driven by a highly conserved set of regulatory genes that operate within transcription–translation feedback loops (TTFLs). These genes and their protein products form the core of the oscillatory mechanism:

1. Period genes (PER1, PER2, and PER3) encode proteins that are central to the negative feedback loop, regulating the timing of circadian cycles.
2. Cryptochrome genes (CRY1 and CRY2) work in concert with PER proteins to inhibit their own transcription, reinforcing rhythmicity.
3. Nuclear receptor subfamily 1 genes—Nr1d1 (REV-ERBα) and Nr1f2 (RORβ or RORγ) function as transcriptional repressors or activators, linking the molecular clock to metabolic regulation.
4. Circadian locomotor output cycles kaput (CLOCK) and NPAS2 encode transcription factors essential for initiating the transcription of core clock genes.
5. Aryl hydrocarbon receptor nuclear translocator-like genes (BMAL1 and BMAL2) form heterodimers with CLOCK or NPAS2 to drive rhythmic transcription of PER and CRY genes.

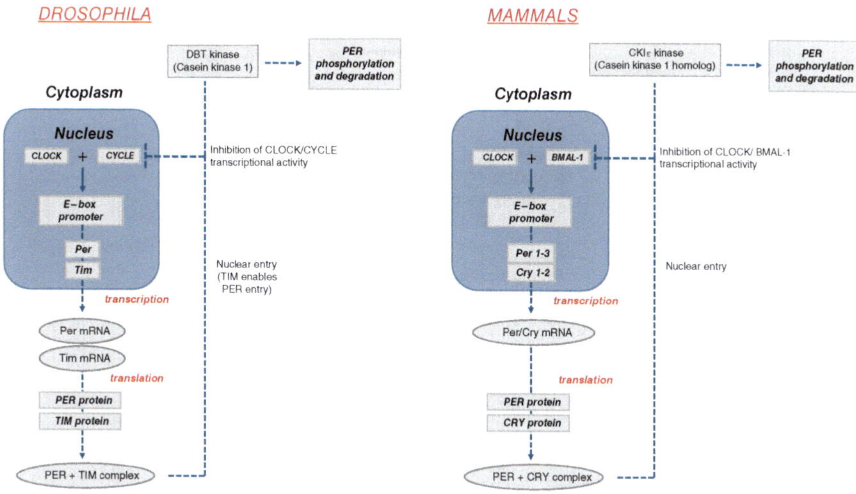


**Fig. 6.2** Simplified representation showing the transcriptional translational feedback loop (TTFL) in different species [4–30]

Together, these regulatory elements establish the rhythmic gene expression patterns that sustain circadian oscillations at the cellular level and synchronize them across tissues. A simplified representation of the transcription–translation feedback loops in drosophila and mammals has been shown in Fig. 6.2.

The PER and CRY proteins enter the cell nucleus where they act as repressors for their own genes' transcription. This step along with the phosphorylation and degradation of PER leads to a delay (−24 h) in the transcriptional translational feedback loop (TTFL) and helps reset the daily cycle. Figure 6.3 demonstrates how core clock genes and transcriptional feedback loops together direct rhythms in a "circadian" fashion.

Transcriptional activators CLOCK, neuronal PAS domain protein 2 (NPAS2), and BMAL1 activate PER and CRY genes to form (CLOCK–BMAL1 and NPAS2–BMAL1). These complexes bind to E-box elements in gene promoters, driving rhythmic PER and CRY transcription, which peaks during the subjective night in the SCN. The resulting PER and CRY proteins translocate to the nucleus, where they inhibit their own transcription, forming the primary negative transcription–translation feedback loop (TTFL) that resets each circadian cycle. A secondary loop enhances rhythm stability through nuclear receptor subfamily 1 group D member 1 (NR1D1/REV-ERB) and retinoic acid receptor-related orphan receptor (ROR) families. Activated by the core oscillator [32], these transcription factors regulate BMAL1 expression via ROR response elements (ROREs), with RORs promoting and REV-ERBs repressing transcription. The primary TTFL and secondary loops work together to sustain the autonomous ~24-h rhythmicity.

The generation of circadian rhythms is dependent on the underlying gene expression. Practically all types of cells (e.g., fibroblasts, myocytes, and

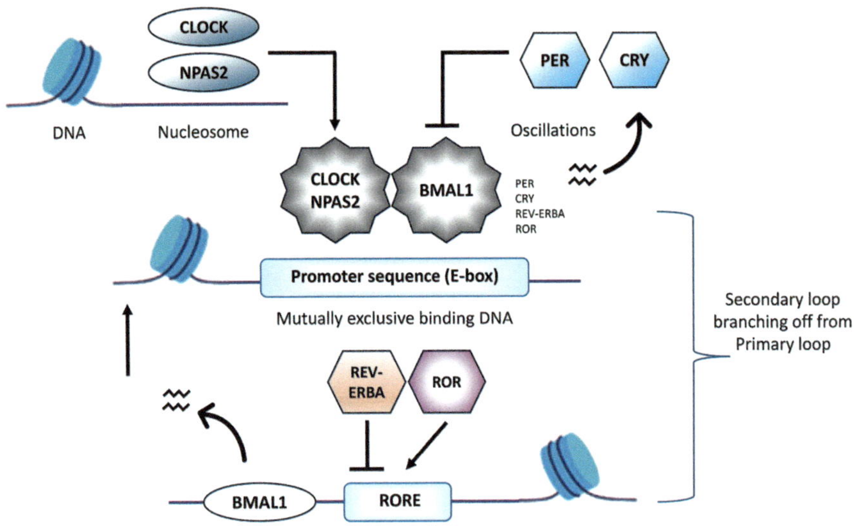


**Fig. 6.3** Core clock genes and transcriptional feedback loops together direct rhythms occurring with a ~24-h periodicity, called "circadian" [3, 31]. Transcription activators, such as CLOCK, NPAS2, and BMAL1, activate PER and CRY gene. The resulting pairs such as CLOCK–BMAL1 and NPAS2–BMAL1 then attach to E-box elements in a specific promoter site, for transcription of PER and CRY genes. The PER and CRY proteins enter the cell nucleus where they act as repressors for their own genes' transcription. This step resets the daily cycle. A secondary feedback loop which includes nuclear receptors belonging to the Nuclear Receptor Subfamily NR1D1, commonly known as REV-ERBA and RAR-Related Orphan Receptor (ROR), is then recruited by components of the core clock oscillator. This leads to the expression of BMAL1 from sites known as ROR response element binding sites (RORE binding sites), circadian locomotor output cycles kaput (CLOCK), neuronal Per-ARNT-Sim domain protein 2 (NPAS2), aryl hydrocarbon receptor nuclear translocator-like protein 1 (ARNTL1, commonly known as BMAL1), period (PER) gene, and cryptochrome gene (CRY) [4–30]

adipocytes) and organs possess an intrinsic oscillatory mechanism. These are termed as peripheral clocks. These cellular and organ-based clocks require coordination into meaningful temporal patterns. The process of coordinating the peripheral clocks is directed by the master circadian pacemaker. This synchronizes the peripheral rhythms in a coherent manner with the key behavioral and physiological cycles. Just like the circadian pacemaker, the peripheral circadian rhythms are also assessed through gene expression in peripheral cells. Even though circadian gene expression is strong, inputs from the suprachiasmatic nucleus, which is composed of clock cells regulated by a transcriptional–translational feedback loop, are essential. Thus, rhythmic gene expression is driven both by intrinsic oscillators and by SCN-mediated extracellular cues, together ensuring optimal physiological function.

### 6.3.2 Regulation of Gene Signaling Pathways

Environmental cues are detected by input gene products, such as melanopsin (an opsin-family photopigment first identified in the inner retina) and RAB3A (identified through mutagenesis screens). These signals are then relayed to the central oscillator which causes reset, synchronization, or entrainment of circadian clock. Specialized photoreceptors regulate the circadian clock and are expressed as proteins that differ in origin, properties, and functions.

The propagation of rhythmic signals to downstream physiological systems is brought about by the output gene products, or *clock-controlled genes*, and includes peptides and transcription factors.

A complex molecular machinery of clock factors maintains the central oscillator to regulate rhythmic expression not only of core clock genes but also of numerous downstream targets. At its core, the molecular circadian mechanism consists of transcriptional–translational feedback loops (TTFLs) involving both positive and negative regulatory elements. These loops generate highly precise 24-h rhythms that govern metabolic processes (e.g., glucose and lipid metabolism), endocrine outputs (e.g., melatonin and corticosteroids), and behavioral rhythms (e.g., feeding and sleep–wake cycle).

### 6.3.3 Importance of the Sleep-Wake Cycle in Human Physiology

A concrete example of genetic influence on circadian rhythms is *chronotype*, the individual preference for sleep–wake timing. Evening chronotype (delayed circadian phase) has been associated with the 3111C allele of the CLOCK gene, whereas morning chronotype (advanced circadian phase) is linked to polymorphisms in PER1, PER2, and PER3. However, more recent evidence indicates that chronotype can be modified by socio-environmental influences. Thus, chronotype reflects an interaction of genetic, environmental, and social determinants, underscoring that circadian rhythmicity emerges from intertwined genetic, physiological, and behavioral mechanisms.

The circadian clock, endocrine system, and peripheral clocks form a well-connected and well-organized regulatory system. The circadian clock regulates the endocrine system, which, in turn, synchronizes and regulates the peripheral clocks [32]. Two types of hormones, *Glucocorticoids* and *Melatonin*, influence the circadian clock for the hierarchal control of the endocrine system and the peripheral clocks.

## 6.4 Pineal Gland: Neuroendocrine Sensor and Actuator

The anatomical relationships of the human pineal gland closely resemble those observed in lower mammals. In lower vertebrates, the pineal gland retains intrinsic photoreceptive capabilities. In contrast, in mammals, it has lost direct photosensitivity and has differentiated into a purely neuroendocrine organ. Neuroanatomical investigations have demonstrated that photic information is transmitted to the pineal gland via a complex, multisynaptic retinohypothalamic–pineal pathway [33–36].

### 6.4.1 Location and Gross Anatomy

Situated in the posterior cranial fossa of the brain, the pineal gland—also known as the *epiphysis cerebri*—is a pine cone-shaped, unpaired structure measuring approximately 0.8 cm in length and weighing around 0.1 g in adults. It is located between the thalamic bodies, just behind the habenular commissure. The gland is in contact with two recesses of the third ventricle: the pineal recess proper and the dorsal suprapineal recess, the latter of which contains the choroid plexus. Positioned near the corpora quadrigemina and posterior to the third ventricle, the pineal gland is bathed in cerebrospinal fluid (CSF) via these recesses [33, 37, 38].

The pineal gland (epiphysis cerebri) occupies a central position in the brain and demonstrates distinct relations in coronal and sagittal sections [39]. On coronal section, it lies inferior to the splenium of the corpus callosum, superior to the inferior and superior colliculi, and superolateral to the choroid plexus of the third ventricle. In sagittal section, it is related anterosuperiorly to the thalamus and the habenular commissure, anteroinferiorly to the cerebral aqueduct of Sylvius, the posterior commissure, and the cerebral peduncle, posterosuperiorly to the cerebral vein of Galen, and inferiorly to the quadrigeminal plate. The gland is richly innervated, receiving adrenergic nerve supply that renders its neurons highly sensitive to epinephrine. Sympathetic fibers arise from the superior cervical ganglion, while parasympathetic inputs are derived from the optic and pterygopalatine ganglia. Additional innervation is contributed by fibers within the pineal stalk, including those originating from neurons of the trigeminal ganglion; these fibers contain the neuropeptide pituitary adenylyl cyclase-activating polypeptide (PACAP). Vascular supply is provided by choroidal branches of the posterior cerebral artery, and venous drainage occurs through the internal cerebral vein. The pia mater forms a capsule and sends septa inward into the gland to form lobules and convey blood vessels into the parenchyma.

Histologically, the pineal gland is composed of two types of cells: pinealocytes and supporting cells. Pinealocytes are specialized neuroendocrine cells with long cytoplasmic processes that extend toward capillaries. These processes help in the release of melatonin and related indoleamines from the pinealocytes directly into the circulation. The activity of these cells is affected by environmental light–dark cycles via sympathetic control. Supporting cells, present in the interstitium, are astrocytic in nature. They provide structural stability and metabolic support.

A characteristic feature of the pineal gland is the presence of corpora arenacea, or "brain sand," which are mineral deposits that progressively accumulate into the gland with age. They appear as calcified bodies and are radiopaque, serving as important landmarks during imaging. The deposits consist of calcium phosphate, magnesium phosphate, calcium carbonate, and ammonium phosphate in varying proportions. The presence of brain sand does not affect pineal gland function.

Pineal gland is the major source of melatonin, a hormone that regulates circadian rhythms and synchronizes peripheral clocks with the central pacemaker in the suprachiasmatic nucleus. Melatonin secretion from the gland follows a circadian pattern, with peak levels at night, thereby serving as a neuroendocrine signal of darkness. In addition, melatonin also exerts regulatory influences on glucose homeostasis, insulin secretion, and energy balance, highlighting its integrative role at the interface of the nervous, endocrine, and metabolic systems.

### 6.4.2 Development and Aging

The pineal gland develops from the lower end of the roof of the third ventricle. By seventh week of intrauterine life, the ependymal region of the roof of third ventricular undergoes thickening and subsequently gives rise to a cavity. Within the cavity, parenchymal cells proliferate to form tubular structures. These cellular tubules differentiate into pinealocytes which are separated by connective tissue and accompanied by developing innervation. The gland continues to mature throughout the first 2 years of age. During this period, the gland acquires a lobular architecture, in which clusters of pinealocytes are divided by connective tissue septa containing blood vessels. The pineal gland reaches a relatively mature form during the first decade of life, and its size thereafter remains stable from approximately 2–20 years of age.

Melatonin levels vary throughout the day and during the lifespan of an individual. Relatively low levels are maintained during daytime, while high levels are maintained at night (typical pattern of diurnal secretion). In newborns, melatonin is detectable in very little quantities and gradually rises. By the age of 6 months, diurnal rhythm is fully established. Nocturnal melatonin concentration increases with a lifetime peak between 4 and 8 years age, following which the levels reduce. Levels decrease most significantly around puberty and remain stable until 40 years of age. Subsequently, the nocturnal concentration declines gradually, and by 70 years of age the levels are comparable to daytime concentration.

## 6.5 Melatonin

In 1958, Lerner's [40] scientific report described the isolation and characterization of melatonin, a compound from the pineal gland of cows (beef pineal glands). Lerner's report was building on the observation that melatonin induced pigment lightening in animals. Before his discovery, for more than four decades, researchers had noted that pineal gland extracts could produce skin lightening in amphibians such as frogs and fish. These extract worked by making melanin granules in skin cells (melanocytes) clump together, which makes the skin appear lighter. This was the opposite of what melanocyte-stimulating hormone (MSH) does—MSH darkens the skin by dispersing melanin. Lerner's objective was to isolate and purify the compound, for which he proposed the name melatonin. The extraction and purification process involved sequential fat removal with petroleum ether, aqueous and ethyl acetate extraction, counter current distribution (ethyl acetate–heptane–water), further solvent extraction and sublimation, and separation by paper chromatography. A distinct blue spot seen on chromatography was visualized using Ehrlich's reagent, indicated the presence of an indole derivative. It resulted in lightening of frog skin which was previously darkened with caffeine. The biological activity of the spot was measured photometrically. It was found to have a strong biological activity, accounting for 95% of the total biological activity of the entire pineal extract. It was found to be highly potent, almost 100 times more potent than adrenaline or noradrenaline in preventing skin darkening, about 200-fold more potent than triiodothyronine, and 5000 times more potent than serotonin. It did not mimic the effects of adrenaline, noradrenaline, or serotonin when tested in other tissues like rat uterus and clam heart, demonstrating that its effects were specific for skin pigmentation. No melatonin was detected in other beef organs like the pituitary, hypothalamus, adrenals, reproductive organs, or eye.

### 6.5.1 Synthesis, Regulation, and Function

Melatonin is a hormone predominantly secreted by the pineal gland. The gland also secretes other substances like biogenic amines, peptides, and γ-aminobutyric acid (GABA). The regulation and secretion of the hormone melatonin is influenced by light–dark cycle. It is exclusively secreted in darkness. The levels of the hormone are not affected by behavioral activity. It shows similar secretory patterns in all animals. Acting as an output signal of the circadian system, melatonin provides feedback to the central clock located in the suprachiasmatic nucleus (SCN) and contributes to the synchronization of both central and peripheral oscillators.

### 6.5.2 Biochemical Pathway of Synthesis

Environmental light, in the retinal photoreceptors, is transduced into electrical signals that are conveyed to the suprachiasmatic nucleus (SCN) primarily through the retinohypothalamic tract (RHT). This pathway is the principal route for mediating light–dark entrainment of the SCN, allowing it to interpret day length and photoperiod. A smaller proportion of visual input reaches the SCN via an alternate route through the primary optic tract and lateral geniculate body, further contributing to circadian regulation [38, 41].

Different wavelengths of light vary in their capacity to entrain circadian rhythms through the suprachiasmatic nucleus (SCN), with yellow–green light being the most effective [38]. Each SCN receives bilateral retinal input, predominantly from the contralateral side, as most fibers cross at the optic chiasm. The ventral and lateral regions of the SCN are the most densely innervated. From the SCN, synaptic connections extend into the lateral hypothalamus and, via the medial forebrain bundle of the brainstem, project downward to the intermediolateral cell column of the spinal cord. Here, preganglionic fibers synapse with the superior cervical ganglion (SCG). Postganglionic noradrenergic fibers then travel through the Nervi conarii, passing across the tentorium cerebelli to innervate the pineal gland [38, 42].

In the absence of light, norepinephrine is released from these postganglionic sympathetic terminals and binds to β-adrenergic receptors on pinealocytes. This leads to activation of adenylyl cyclase and increase in intracellular cyclic adenosine monophosphate (cAMP) levels. Elevated cAMP initiates a series of downstream signaling cascades. There is activation of catalytic subunits of protein kinase A and phosphorylation of the cAMP response element-binding protein (CREB). Since cAMP response elements (CREs) are present in the promoter region of the arylalkylamine N-acetyltransferase (AANAT) gene, this pathway drives increased transcription of the enzyme arylalkylamine N-acetyltransferase. It is the rate-limiting enzyme in melatonin synthesis. Consequently, the absence of light regulates melatonin production through sympathetic neural pathways, producing the characteristic circadian rhythm of melatonin secretion [33, 43].

Melatonin synthesis (Fig. 6.4) begins with tryptophan, an essential amino acid. It undergoes the following sequential enzymatic steps in the pineal gland:

1. Hydroxylation—of tryptophan by the enzyme tryptophan hydroxylase to produce 5-hydroxytryptophan
2. Decarboxylation—of 5-hydroxytryptophan by aromatic-L-amino acid decarboxylase to give serotonin (5-hydroxytryptamine, 5-HT)
3. Acetylation (rate-limiting step)—of serotonin by aralkylamine N-acetyltransferase (AANAT) to produce N-acetylserotonin. This step represents the major regulatory point in melatonin biosynthesis.
4. Methylation—of N-acetylserotonin at the 5-hydroxy position by hydroxyindole-O-methyltransferase (HIOMT, also known as acetylserotonin O-methyltransferase, ASMT) to yield melatonin

### 6.5.3 Regulation by Light and Circadian Control

The synthesis and secretion of melatonin are under circadian control. The activity of aralkylamine N-acetyltransferase (AANAT) is the major regulatory point in melatonin biosynthesis. The expression of AANAT and melatonin synthesis and secretion follow daily rhythmic patterns. Darkness acts as the primary signal for biosynthesis of melatonin. Exposure to light at during night suppresses the expression of AANAT and terminates melatonin synthesis and release.

This is regulated via a well-defined neural pathway. Light is detected by retinal photoreceptors and transmitted to the suprachiasmatic nucleus. The SCN projects to the pineal gland via a complex pathway involving the sympathetic nervous system. Melatonin is then secreted from the pineal gland providing a reliable hormonal reflection of the light–dark cycle. It helps encode for the night length and provides information regarding the environmental photoperiod.

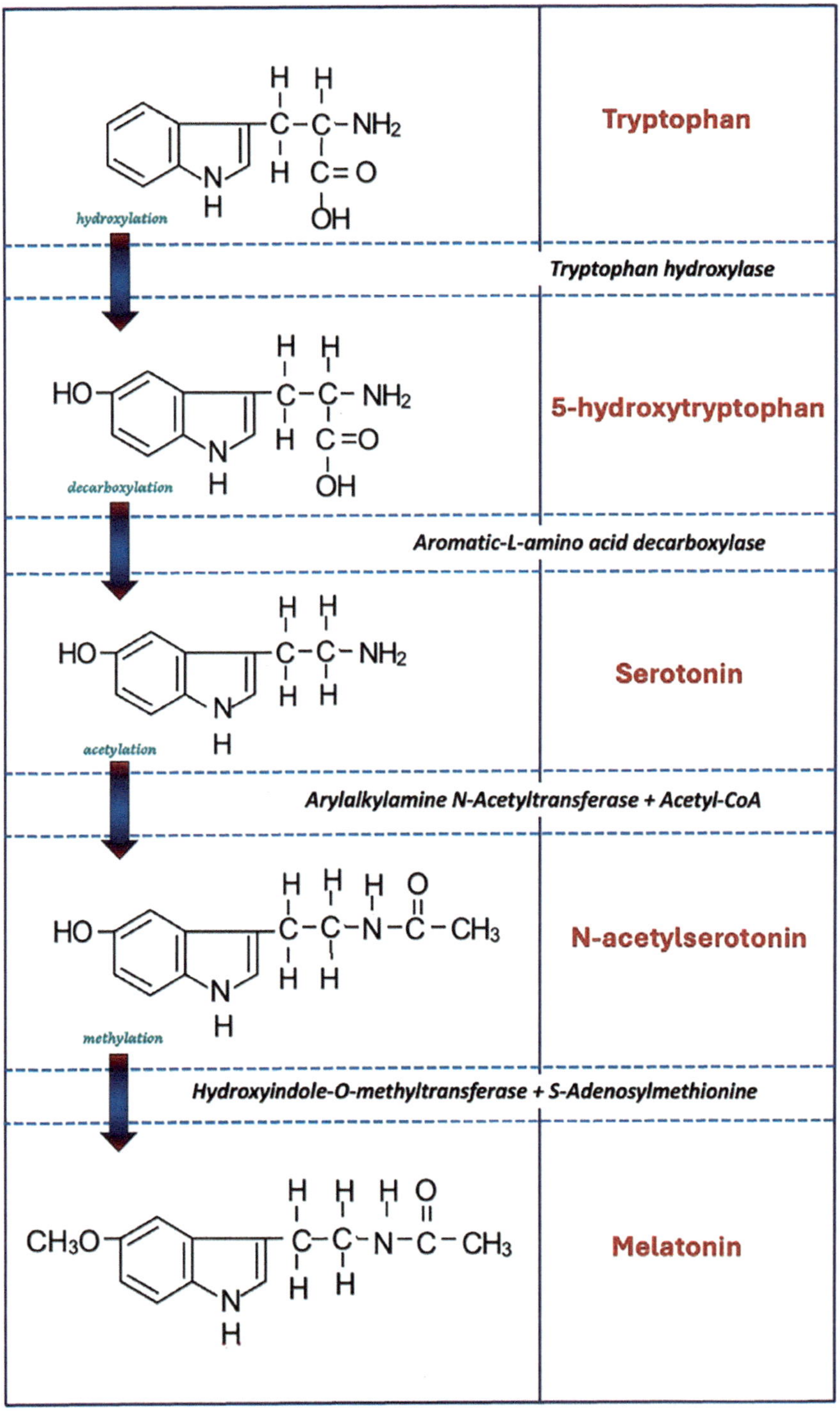


**Fig. 6.4** Melatonin biosynthesis [42, 43]

### 6.5.4 Secretion and Metabolism

Melatonin, as compared to the other hormones, is not stored in significant quantities within the pineal gland. It is synthesized and released immediately into the bloodstream and the cerebrospinal fluid. Plasma concentrations of melatonin reflect pineal activity with maximum rise during the night in direct proportion to the aralkylamine N-acetyltransferase activity.

Melatonin undergoes rapid metabolism in the liver and has a short half-life of a few minutes. It undergoes 6-hydroxylation followed by conjugation in the liver and is subsequently excreted via the kidneys. The synthesis, secretion, and rapid clearance of melatonin mirror the real-time environmental light–dark conditions.

Various factors determine whether a specific light stimulus can regulate melatonin secretion in humans.

- Size, brightness, and spectral quality of light source
- Gaze behavior relative to light source
- Age of the ocular lens
- Pupillary dilatation
- Sensitivity of operative photopigments and photoreceptors
- Photoreceptor in the retina
- Ability of circadian system to integrate photic stimuli spatially and temporally

Figure 6.5 shows various physiological factors that control pineal hormone secretion and its delivery to target organs.

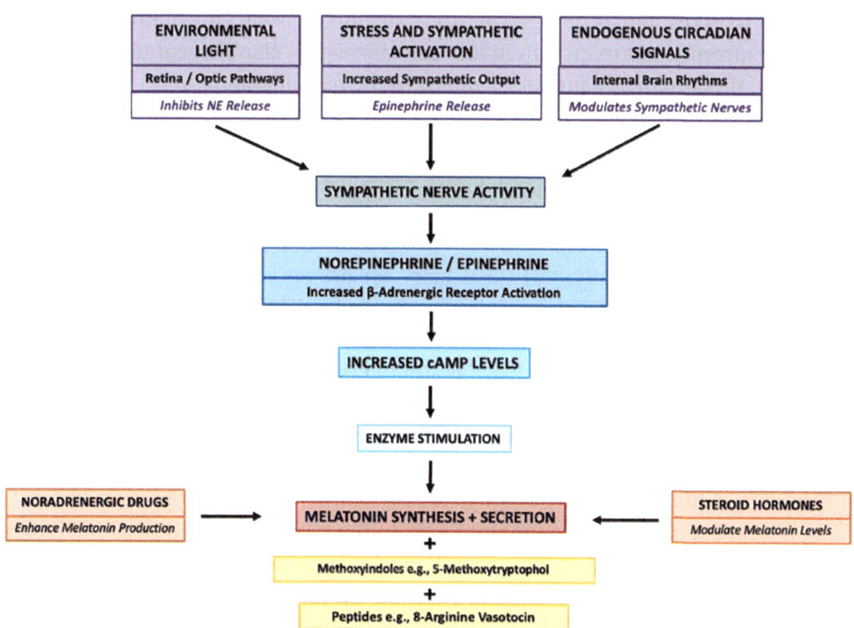


**Fig. 6.5** Schematic diagram to show the factors controlling pineal hormone secretion and delivery to target organs [42, 43]

### 6.5.5 Physiological Roles of Melatonin

Melatonin serves as a hormonal signal of darkness. It plays a major role in central clock mechanisms, helps to synchronize peripheral oscillators, and conveys photoperiodic information that is essential for diurnal and seasonal physiology.

In addition to circadian regulation, melatonin also plays a role in regulation of the reproductive axis, particularly in seasonal breeders. Melatonin, in seasonal breeders, affects fertility, puberty, and gonadal activity.

### 6.5.6 Circadian and Systemic Actions

Melatonin acts on the suprachiasmatic nucleus, the central circadian pacemaker, leading to a reduction in the neuronal firing of SCN and thereby causing clock entrainment. It simultaneously coordinates circadian oscillators in the peripheral tissues, to ensure temporal alignment across all organ systems. It helps encode the duration of night to provide the organism with an internal representation of day length. This representation serves as a signal that is critical for diurnal and seasonal adjustments in physiology and behavior.

### 6.5.7 Melatonin and Reproduction

Experimental studies done on rodents and sheep have demonstrated that removal of the pineal gland leads to precocious puberty. Studies have also revealed that exposure to light and prolonged periods of darkness or enucleation results in testicular atrophy and reduction in the testosterone levels. These findings suggest the role of melatonin as a potent regulator of the hypothalamic–pituitary–gonadal (HPG) axis.

The significance of melatonin in reproductive physiology is most evident in seasonal breeders, wherein the reproductive capacity is tightly linked to amount of photoperiod. In these species, melatonin secretion serves as a temporal signal that aligns reproductive activity with environmental conditions affecting fertility, puberty, and gonadal activity. It also helps ensure survival of the offspring. For example, in sheep and horses, the timing of reproductive cycles helps to ensure that gestation coincides with favorable seasons. The direction of melatonin's influence varies between species. The influence is stimulatory in some species whereas inhibitory in others.

Melatonin regulates reproductive health via precise neuroendocrine signaling.

- Melatonin duration acts as a signal: The nocturnal duration of melatonin secretion conveys photoperiodic information to the pars tuberalis, where melatonin binds to MT1 receptors expressed at high density.
- Production of TSHβ: Activation of MT1 influences the expression of clockwork proteins such as Cry1, which modulate the production of thyroid-stimulating hormone β (TSHβ).

- Tanycyte response: TSHβ acts locally on tanycytes, specialized glial cells in the mediobasal hypothalamus, by binding to TSH receptors on them. This interaction regulates the expression of type 2 (D2) and type 3 (D3) iodothyronine deiodinases, to control the local bioavailability of thyroid hormone (T3).
- Under long-day conditions resulting in short melatonin duration, D2 expression is upregulated. This results in an increase in the local bioavailability of T3 in the mediobasal hypothalamus, resulting in reproductive activation.
- Under short-day conditions resulting in long melatonin duration, D3 expression predominates, reducing T3 levels and leading to reproductive suppression.

Experimental evidence shows that administration of T3 into the hypothalamus of short-day animals is sufficient to restore reproductive function, underscoring the critical role of thyroid hormone signaling in this pathway.

### 6.5.8 Thyroid Hormone and GnRH Regulation

The downstream effects of thyroid hormone involve secretion of gonadotropin-releasing hormone (GnRH). End-feet of tanycytes ensheathe GnRH axon terminals in the median eminence. The position of the end-feet is under the influence of T3 hormone. When the levels of T3 increase, these end-foot processes retract. This releases the GnRH terminals which then reach the fenestrated portal vessels. They stimulate gonadotropin release from the anterior pituitary. Apart from tanycyte-mediated GnRH release, thyroid hormone receptors are widely distributed throughout the hypothalamus and regulate the expression of kisspeptin, a peptide critical for pulsatile GnRH release.

## 6.6 Melatonin Receptors and Mechanisms of Action

Melatonin acts via specific melatonin receptors as well as through direct molecular interactions. The physiological effects of melatonin include but are limited to circadian regulation, glucose homeostasis, antioxidant, and anticancer potential [33, 43].

### 6.6.1 Melatonin Receptors

Melatonin exerts its action primarily through G protein-coupled receptors (GPCRs). Two types of G protein-coupled receptors for melatonin have been identified: MT1 (or Mel1a) and MT2 (or Mel1b). MT1 receptor is a high-affinity receptor. It was first identified in Xenopus melanophores. It is widely expressed in the human body, particularly in the suprachiasmatic nucleus, retina, and the pars tuberalis. MT2 receptor shares ~60% homology with MT1. It is expressed at lower levels in the

SCN and retina and is thought to mediate phase-shifting effects of melatonin. A third category of melatonin receptor, MT3, is not a G protein-coupled receptor, but a high-affinity binding site located on quinone reductase 2, a cytosolic detoxification enzyme. MT3 binding may explain some of melatonin's antioxidant and cytoprotective properties. In addition to receptor-mediated effects, melatonin also functions as a direct free radical scavenger, neutralizing reactive oxygen and reactive nitrogen species.

### 6.6.2 Melatonin and Circadian Regulation

In the SCN, melatonin reduces neuronal activity, thereby modulating the master pacemaker. This inhibitory action is primarily mediated through MT1 receptors, as shown by genetic knockout studies: Deletion of MT1 abolishes melatonin's inhibitory effects on SCN neurons, while deletion of MT2 does not. Conversely, phase-shifting effects of melatonin appear to depend more strongly on MT2 signaling.

These findings suggest that:

- MT1 → inhibition of SCN neuronal firing
- MT2 → phase-shifting of circadian rhythms

This neuroanatomic specificity is supported by the distribution of melatonin receptor mRNA, which overlaps with radiolabeled melatonin binding sites in circadian regulatory regions.

Melatonin also influences the expression of core clock genes, thereby modulating circadian molecular machinery. For example, removal of the MT2 receptor decreases Per1 and Cry1 expression in the SCN. In cell studies, melatonin treatment has been shown to increase Per1 and CLOCK, while reducing BMAL1 expression, although most of this work has been in cancer models and requires extension to normal tissues.

In turn, circadian genes may regulate melatonin synthesis and action. For instance, Per1 knockout (KO) mice display elevated melatonin during the active phase, raising the possibility that disrupted feedback contributes to altered insulin secretion. Knockdown of CLOCK or BMAL1 could hypothetically upregulate melatonin, supporting a bidirectional relationship between clock genes and melatonin signaling.

### 6.6.3 Melatonin and Glucose Homeostasis

Experimental studies on the role of melatonin in metabolic regulation suggest that melatonin may inhibit glucose-stimulated insulin secretion (GSIS). This has led to hypotheses connecting melatonin signaling with diabetes pathophysiology.

- In humans, a genetic association has been identified between a single nucleotide polymorphism (SNP) near the MTNR1B gene (encoding MT2) and increased fasting glucose, as well as greater incidence of type 2 diabetes in both European and Asian populations.

- A clinical study compared the plasma melatonin levels in three cohorts: lean men, obese nondiabetic men, and obese type 2 diabetic men. It was observed that the obese nondiabetic men had higher plasma melatonin and leptin levels than the other two groups. The physiological significance of this finding remains unclear.

### 6.6.4 Anticarcinogenic Potential

Beyond circadian and metabolic regulation, melatonin has been shown to have anticarcinogenic potential. Treatment with melatonin has been shown to alter the clock gene expression resulting in antiproliferative effects in prostate tumor cells, resulting in tumor suppression.

The Nobel Prize in Physiology or Medicine was awarded in 2017 to researchers who identified the molecular mechanisms governing circadian rhythms. They used fruit flies as a model organism to isolate a gene that controls the normal daily biological rhythm. The gene was found to encode a protein that accumulated in the cell during the night and is then degraded during the day. Subsequently, they identified additional protein components of the machinery, to decode the mechanism governing the self-sustaining clock in the cell [4].

## References

1. Kappers JA. Short history of pineal discovery and research. In: Progress in brain research [Internet]. Elsevier; 1979 [cited 2025 Aug 28]. p. 3–22. Available from: https://linkinghub.elsevier.com/retrieve/pii/S0079612308629088.
2. Kuhlman SJ, Craig LM, Duffy JF. Introduction to chronobiology. Cold Spring Harb Perspect Biol. 2018;10(9):a033613.
3. Morin R, Forest G, Imbeault P. Circadian rhythms revealed: unraveling the genetic, physiological, and behavioral tapestry of the human biological clock and rhythms. Front Sleep. 2025;4:1544945.
4. Huang RC. The discoveries of molecular mechanisms for the circadian rhythm: the 2017 Nobel Prize in Physiology or Medicine. Biom J. 2018;41(1):5–8.
5. Ibáñez C. The 2017 Nobel Prize in Physiology or Medicine—advanced information: discoveries of molecular mechanisms controlling the circadian rhythm. Nobelprize.org. Nobel Media AB; 2014. Available from: http://www.nobelprize.org/nobel_prizes/medicine/laureates/2017/advanced.html.
6. Rosbash M. A 50-year personal journey: location, gene expression, and circadian rhythms. Cold Spring Harb Perspect Biol. 2017;9:a032516.
7. Bargiello TA, Young MW. Molecular genetics of a biological clock in Drosophila. Proc Natl Acad Sci U S A. 1984;81:2142–6.
8. Bargiello TA, Jackson FR, Young MW. Restoration of circadian behavioural rhythms by gene transfer in Drosophila. Nature. 1984;312:752–4.
9. Reddy P, Zehring WA, Wheeler DA, Pirrotta V, Hadfield C, Hall JC, et al. Molecular analysis of the period locus in Drosophila melanogaster and identification of a transcript involved in biological rhythms. Cell. 1984;38:701–10.

10. Zehring WA, Wheeler DA, Reddy P, Konopka RJ, Kyriacou CP, Rosbash M, et al. P-element transformation with period locus DNA restores rhythmicity to mutant, arrhythmic Drosophila melanogaster. Cell. 1984;39:369–76.
11. Crews ST, Thomas JB, Goodman CS. The Drosophila single-minded gene encodes a nuclear protein with sequence similarity to the per gene product. Cell. 1988;52:143–52.
12. Siwicki KK, Eastman C, Petersen G, Rosbash M, Hall JC. Antibodies to the period gene product of Drosophila reveal diverse tissue distribution and rhythmic changes in the visual system. Neuron. 1988;1:141–50.
13. Hardin PE, Hall JC, Rosbash M. Feedback of the Drosophila period gene product on circadian cycling of its messenger RNA levels. Nature. 1990;343:536–40.
14. Liu X, Zwiebel LJ, Hinton D, Benzer S, Hall JC, Rosbash M. The period gene encodes a predominantly nuclear protein in adult Drosophila. J Neurosci. 1992;12:2735–44.
15. Zeng H, Hardin PE, Rosbash M. Constitutive overexpression of the Drosophila period protein inhibits period mRNA cycling. EMBO J. 1994;13:3590–8.
16. Myers MP, Wager-Smith K, Wesley CS, Young MW, Sehgal A. Positional cloning and sequence analysis of the Drosophila clock gene timeless. Science. 1995;270:805–8.
17. Sehgal A, Rothenfluh-Hilfiker A, Hunter-Ensor M, Chen Y, Myers MP, Young MW. Rhythmic expression of timeless: a basis for promoting circadian cycles in period gene autoregulation. Science. 1995;270:808–10.
18. Sehgal A, Price J, Man B, Young MW. Loss of circadian behavioral rhythms and per RNA oscillations in the Drosophila mutant timeless. Science. 1994;263:1603–6.
19. Gekakis N, Saez L, Delahaye-Brown A, Myers MP, Sehgal A, Young MW, et al. Isolation of timeless by PER protein interactions: defective interaction between timeless protein and long-period mutant PERL. Science. 1995;270:811–5.
20. Vosshall LB, Price JL, Sehgal A, Saez L, Young MW. Block in nuclear localization of period protein by a second clock mutation, timeless. Science. 1994;263:1606–9.
21. Price JL, Dembinska ME, Young MW, Rosbash M. Suppression of PERIOD protein abundance and circadian cycling by the Drosophila clock mutation timeless. EMBO J. 1995;14:4044–9.
22. Vitaterna MH, King DP, Chang AM, Kornhauser JM, Lowrey PL, McDonald JD, et al. Mutagenesis and mapping of a mouse gene, Clock, essential for circadian behavior. Science. 1994;264:719–25.
23. King DP, Zhao Y, Sangoram AM, Wilsbacher LD, Tanaka M, Antoch MP, et al. Positional cloning of the mouse circadian clock gene. Cell. 1997;89:641–53.
24. Antoch MP, Song EJ, Chang AM, Vitaterna MH, Zhao Y, Wilsbacher LD, et al. Functional identification of the mouse circadian clock gene by transgenic BAC rescue. Cell. 1997;89:655–67.
25. Gekakis N, Staknis D, Nguyen HB, Davis CF, Wilsbacher LD, King DP, et al. Role of the CLOCK protein in the mammalian circadian mechanism. Science. 1998;280:1564–9.
26. Darlington TK, Wager-Smith K, Ceriani MF, Staknis D, Gekakis N, Steeves TD, et al. Closing the circadian feedback loop: CLOCK-induced transcription of its own inhibitors, period and timeless. Science. 1998;280:1599–603.
27. Allada R, White NE, So WV, Hall JC, Rosbash M. A mutant Drosophila homolog of mammalian Clock disrupts circadian rhythms and transcription of period and timeless. Cell. 1998;93:791–804.
28. Rutila JE, Suri V, Le M, So WV, Rosbash M, Hall JC. CYCLE is a second bHLH-PAS clock protein essential for circadian rhythmicity and transcription of Drosophila period and timeless. Cell. 1998;93:805–14.
29. Price JL, Blau J, Rothenfluh A, Abodeely M, Kloss B, Young MW. Double-time is a novel Drosophila clock gene that regulates PERIOD protein accumulation. Cell. 1998;94:83–95.
30. Kloss B, Price JL, Saez L, Blau J, Rothenfluh A, Wesley CS, Young MW, et al. The Drosophila clock gene double-time encodes a protein closely related to human casein kinase Iε. Cell. 1998;94:97–107.
31. Reinke H, Asher G. Crosstalk between metabolism and circadian clocks. Nat Rev Mol Cell Biol. 2019;20(4):227–41.

32. Richards J, Gumz ML. Mechanism of the circadian clock in physiology. Am J Physiol-Regul Integr Comp Physiol. 2013;304(12):R1053–64.
33. Reiter RJ, Tan DX, Galano A. Melatonin: exceeding expectations. Physiology. 2014;29(5):325–33.
34. Reiter RJ. The mammalian pineal gland: structure and function. Am J Anat. 1981;162(4):287–313.
35. Kappers JA. The mammalian pineal gland, a survey. Acta Neurochir (Wien). 1976;34(1–4):109–49.
36. Tapp E. The histology and pathology of the human pineal gland. In: Progress in brain research [Internet]. Elsevier; 1979 [cited 2025 Aug 28]. p. 481–500. Available from: https://linkinghub.elsevier.com/retrieve/pii/S0079612308629556.
37. Møller M, Baeres FM. The anatomy and innervation of the mammalian pineal gland. Cell Tissue Res. 2002;309(1):139–50.
38. Erlich SS, Apuzzo MLJ. The pineal gland: anatomy, physiology, and clinical significance. J Neurosurg. 1985;63(3):321–41.
39. Ilahi S, Beriwal N, Ilahi TB. Physiology, pineal gland [Updated 2023 Apr 24]. In: StatPearls [Internet]. Treasure Island: StatPearls Publishing; 2025 Jan-. Available from: https://www.ncbi.nlm.nih.gov/books/NBK525955/.
40. Lerner AB, Case JD, Takahashi Y, Lee TH, Mori W. Isolation of melatonin, the pineal gland factor that lightens MELANOCYTES1. J Am Chem Soc. 1958;80(10):–2587. https://doi.org/10.1021/ja01543a060.
41. Moore RY, Klein DC. Visual pathways and the central neural control of a circadian rhythm in pineal serotonin N-acetyltransferase activity. Brain Res. 1974;71(1):17–33.
42. Wurtman RJ, Moskowitz MA. The pineal organ (first of two parts). N Engl J Med. 1977;296(23):1329–33. https://doi.org/10.1056/NEJM197706092962307.
43. Sugden D. Melatonin biosynthesis in the mammalian pineal gland. Experientia. 1989;45(10):922–32.

# Endocrine Control of Metabolism: Hormonal Regulation of Energy Homeostasis

7

Tania Talwar

**Abstract**

Energy homeostasis in the body is maintained by regulating the nutrient intake, energy storage, and energy utilization. This is brought about by the interplay of endocrine, neural, and metabolic pathways. This chapter provides a comprehensive overview of the role of endocrine system in the control of metabolism. Emphasis has been made on the integration of central and peripheral signals governing energy balance in both physiological and pathological states. The hypothalamus functions as a central hub, integrating neurohormonal signals mainly from the gastrointestinal tract, pancreas, liver, and adipose tissue, translating these signals into appropriate endocrine and autonomic response. Adipose tissue, once considered to be a passive energy depot, is now recognized as an active endocrine organ.

This chapter reviews the role of hormones insulin, glucagon, incretins, ghrelin, thyroid hormones, glucocorticoids, and catecholamines in orchestrating anabolic and catabolic states. A particular emphasis has been made on metabolism of lipids, carbohydrates, and proteins by the hormones. Pathophysiological correlates, such as obesity and type 1 and type 2 diabetes mellitus, have also been discussed linking them with lipostat and various programming hypotheses. This chapter highlights the central role of hormonal regulation in maintaining energy homeostasis by integrating various molecular, physiological, and clinical perspectives.

T. Talwar (✉)
Department of Physiology, All India Institute of Medical Sciences, New Delhi, India





H. Prabhakar, M. Kaur (eds.), *Brain and Endocrine Crosstalk*, Physiology in Clinical Neurosciences – Brain and Spinal Cord Crosstalks,
https://doi.org/10.1007/978-981-92-0763-3_7

**Keywords**

Energy homeostasis · Endocrine regulation of metabolism · Adipose tissue · Leptin · Adiponectin · Insulin · Gut hormones · Ghrelin · Incretins · Lipostat · Obesity · Diabetes mellitus · Hypothalamic regulation

## 7.1 Introduction

Humans depend on regular nutrient intake to sustain life. The biological drivers for nutrient ingestion are triggered during states of energy deprivation and turned off with energy provision. These processes are regulated by hormonal and neuroendocrine systems via a network of central and peripheral signals. These networks include mechanisms that are involved in nutrient sensing, signals from organs reflecting their energetic state, and the translation of these signals into actions. Both afferent neural inputs and hormonal signals convey information to the brain, where the signals for hunger and satiety are generated. Through interplay of all these signals and mechanisms, the relationship thus maintained between energy intake, expenditure, and storage is quantified as *energy balance* [1]. The hypothalamus plays a central role in integrating afferent metabolic signals and, in coordination with other regions in the brain, regulates pituitary function to maintain neurohormonal control of metabolism. Through efferent neural and endocrine pathways, the brain influences the different peripheral organs involved in energy homeostasis.

Energy status of an individual undergoes both acute and long-term changes. Acute fluctuations in the energy balance occur daily, while long-term and chronic alterations affect energy reserves and necessitate compensatory adaptations. The fine balance is controlled by an internal set point that senses the quantity of energy stores and regulates food intake and energy expenditure. Reduced energy states and food deprivation, leading to chronic negative energy balance, result in neuroendocrine responses which include but are not limited to suppression of the hypothalamic–pituitary–gonadal and thyroid axes, increased cortisol secretion, enhanced insulin sensitivity, and a reduction in the leptin-to-adiponectin ratio. In contrast, a sustained state of surplus energy restores, leading to chronic positive energy balance, results in restoration of pituitary activity, promotes insulin resistance, and elevates the leptin-to-adiponectin ratio [1–4].

In 1953, Gordon Kennedy [5] proposed the lipostat model in his seminal paper *The Role of Depot Fat in the Hypothalamic Control of Food Intake*. He suggested that adipose tissue functions as a regulatory organ, providing a feedback signal to the hypothalamus to maintain body fat at a stable "set point." In this model, a reduction in fat stores would stimulate hunger and increase food intake, whereas

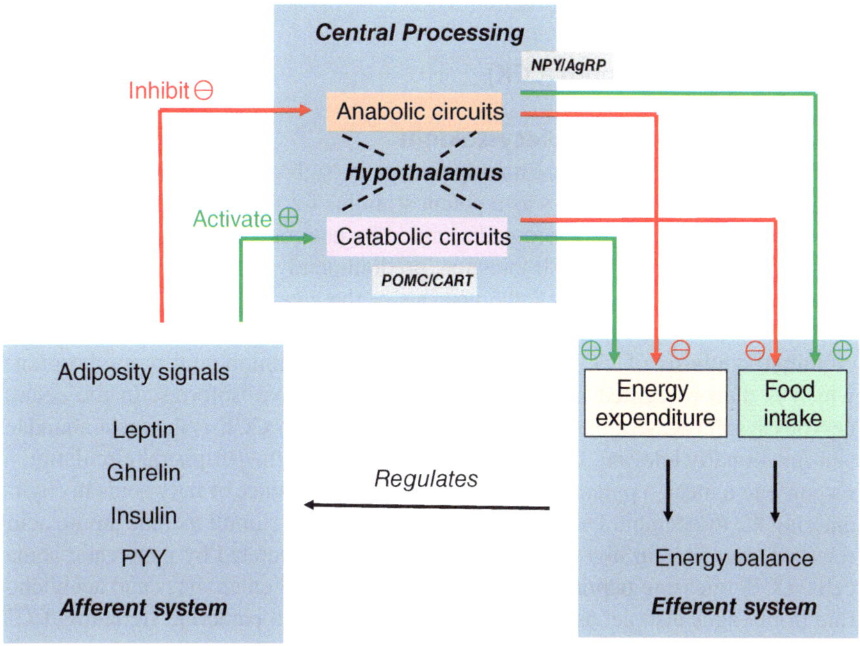


**Fig. 7.1** The fine balance is controlled by an internal set point called the lipostat that senses the quantity of energy stores and regulates food intake and energy expenditure. Components of this energy balance are: Afferent system or peripheral system consisting of leptin, ghrelin, insulin, and PYY; Arcuate nucleus of hypothalamus, which generates the new signals transmitted by POMC/CART(anorexigenic and causes expenditure) or NPY/AgRP(orexigenic and causes food intake); Efferent pathways which are either anabolic or catabolic. *NPY* neuropeptide Y, *AgRP* agouti-related peptide, *PYY* peptide YY, *POMC* proopiomelanocortin, *CART* cocaine and amphetamine-regulated transcript

expansion of fat depots would suppress appetite. Kennedy hypothesized the existence of a circulating humoral factor derived from adipose tissue that communicated the status of fat reserves to the brain, although the identity of this signal was unknown at the time.

Decades later, with the discovery of leptin in 1994, Kennedy's proposal of the lipostat was validated. Leptin is a hormone which is produced by the adipocytes. With an increase in the fat stores, there is a proportional increase in the amount of leptin secreted. Leptin signals the hypothalamus to decrease the amount of food consumed and increase the amount of energy expenditure. The historical progression—from a theoretical model of lipostat to the molecular confirmation of leptin—established the foundation of modern understanding of energy homeostasis and obesity. Figure 7.1 depicts the lipostat control and its various components.

## 7.2 Fat Metabolism

### 7.2.1 Cholecystokinin (CCK)

#### 7.2.1.1 Regulation of Cholecystokinin

Ingested fats after digestion are mainly present in triglyceride form, the presence of which in the duodenum serves as a potent stimulus for the release of cholecystokinin (CCK). CCK is synthesized and secreted by enteroendocrine I cells located in the mucosal lining of the small intestine, predominantly in the duodenum and jejunum. In addition to these sites, the neurons of the enteric nervous system and the brain also secrete CCK [1].

Initial synthesis of CCK is in the form of a 115-amino acid preprohormone, which is then processed into several biologically active isoforms. In the central nervous system (CNS), the sulfated octapeptide form of CCK is the most abundant and functionally relevant. CCK is rapidly released into the peripheral circulation in response to a meal, a potent trigger for which is the presence of fatty acids in chyme entering the duodenum. Other less potent but important stimuli include amino acids released after protein digestion and monitor peptide secreted by pancreatic acinar cells. CCK-releasing peptide from gastric and intestinal enterocytes and acetylcholine from vagus also act as stimuli for CCK release, via paracrine signaling. CCK has a relatively short plasma half-life of about 2.5 min.

Reduction in cholecystokinin (CCK) synthesis and secretion is brought about by decrease in luminal free fatty acids. Other potent inhibitors for CCK release are somatostatin, pancreatic peptide, and trypsin released from the exocrine pancreas. They downregulate the production of CCK by inactivating both CCK-releasing peptide from gastric and intestinal enterocytes and monitor peptide from pancreatic acinar cells.

#### 7.2.1.2 Actions of Cholecystokinin

CCK has a wide range of physiological and neurobehavioral effects. In the gastrointestinal system, CCK increases gastric emptying time and stimulates pancreatic acinar cells via CCK-A receptors to promote the release of digestive enzymes. It also increases bile production and bile secretion by inducing contraction of the gallbladder and biliary tree. In addition, it also brings about the relaxation of the sphincter of Oddi resulting in flow of bile and pancreatic enzymes into the duodenum.

Beyond its gastrointestinal functions, CCK, in its sulfated octapeptide form, plays a crucial role in the central nervous system. Activation of its receptors contributes to the regulation of satiety, while stimulation of CCK-B receptors in various CNS centers induces anxiety. Moreover, the CCK tetrapeptide fragment can precipitate panic responses by activating neurons within the anterior cingulate cortex, vermis of the cerebellum, and the claustro-amygdaloid complex.

#### 7.2.1.3 Digestion, Absorption, and Transport of Lipids

Dietary triglycerides are digested by the coordinated action of pancreatic lipases and intestinal lipases. These enzymes hydrolyze lipids step by step, initially removing one fatty acid chain from the triglycerides to form diglycerides. This is followed by further hydrolysis and cleaving of another fatty acid to give monoglycerides. In the final step, a complete breakdown of monoglyceride releases glycerol and free fatty acid. These free fatty acids are then emulsified into micelles by the action of bile acids. Micelles facilitate lipid absorption across the intestinal brush border mucosa, thereby enabling the delivery of glycerol and free fatty acids (FFAs) into enterocytes. Within the enterocytes, there is reesterification of the absorbed glycerol and free fatty acids to form new triglyceride (TG) molecules which are then assembled into lipoprotein particles. Apolipoprotein B48 serves as the structural backbone for this assembly, resulting in the formation of chylomicrons, the primary carriers of dietary lipids in the circulation. These chylomicrons then move into the mesenteric lymphatic vessels and via the thoracic duct enter the venous circulation. During the transit, they bypass the liver, resulting in no first-pass metabolism. The first major capillary network that the chylomicrons encounter is in the lungs. Subsequent to this, they enter the left atrium and the left ventricle, finally to be distributed via the systemic circulation to the peripheral tissues, including the liver.

#### 7.2.1.4 Storage and Mobilization of Lipids

Triglycerides are transported in the form of chylomicrons to adipose tissues, the principal reservoir for energy storage in the form of fat. The storage process is a hallmark of the anabolic state where energy substrates are directed toward building and conserving the reserves. Genetic differences can influence the distribution of fat across various parts of the body; however, with continuous fat mobilization and storage, an increase in adipose tissue mass occurs in all depots, irrespective of their location. In majority of the individuals, the intra-abdominal fat stores represent the predominant site of storage.

Within the adipocytes, triglyceride storage in lipid vacuoles is under tight control of hormones. β-adrenergic receptor activation and epinephrine release accelerate the movement of long-chain fatty acids (LCFAs) across the plasma membrane, increasing transport rates up to five to ten times above normal. The underlying mechanism involves cAMP-mediated activation of hormone-sensitive lipase, thus driving lipolysis. Insulin, however, exerts an opposing effect, completely abolishing the lipolytic response to epinephrine in physiological concentrations. Insulin role in regulation of LCFA transport influences both influx and efflux, thereby counteracting lipolysis, suppressing lipid mobilization, and promoting lipogenesis. This balance between epinephrine-driven mobilization and insulin-driven storage illustrates the endocrine regulation of the transition between catabolic and anabolic states.

Triglycerides in the form of chylomicrons are also transported to the liver via the arterial circulation. Excessive delivery of saturated fats leads to hepatosteatosis and increases the secretion of very low-density lipoprotein (VLDL). Omega-3 fatty acids, however, exert opposing and protective effect, reducing hepatosteatosis and lowering the hepatic VLDL secretion.

During fasting, a classical example of catabolic state, adipocytes release the stored fatty acids into the circulation via increased activity of hormone-sensitive lipase. These fatty acids in the circulation undergo β-oxidation to produce acetyl-CoA, which then enters the citric acid cycle in hepatocytes, myocytes, and certain other tissues (e.g., kidney, brain, and immune cells) to sustain energy production in the absence of exogenous nutrient supply.

#### 7.2.1.5 Endocrine Role of Adipose Tissue

White adipose tissue (WAT), originally considered as energy storage depot, is now widely recognized and considered as an active endocrine organ that plays a central role in regulation of energy homeostasis and metabolic functions. This modern view builds directly on Kennedy's lipostat model (1953), which proposed that fat stores provide feedback signals to the hypothalamus to regulate appetite and body weight. With the discovery of leptin in 1994, further evidence of adipose tissue as a critical communicator in energy balance rather than merely a storage site was provided [6].

##### Major Adipokines

- Leptin: It is secreted in proportion to fat mass. It acts via the hypothalamus to suppress appetite and increase overall energy expenditure. In cases of obesity, there is increased leptin resistance. The overall effect in obesity is normal or increased appetite and decreased energy expenditure contributing to persistent weight gain [7].
- Adiponectin: It is an adipokine that acts by enhancing insulin sensitivity, increasing fatty acid oxidation, and upregulating the anti-inflammatory effects. In cases of obesity, adiponectin levels decline, leading to metabolic dysfunction.

##### Other Adipokines

- Resistin: associated with insulin resistance; inhibition improves insulin sensitivity [8].
- Visfatin exhibits insulin-mimetic actions, binding to the insulin receptor.
- Omentin-1: reduced in obesity; restored by metformin, with beneficial effects on insulin sensitivity
- Obestatin: downregulated in obesity and type 2 diabetes mellitus (T2DM)
- Retinol-Binding Protein 4 (RBP4): Correlates with insulin resistance severity.
- Asprosin: a WAT-derived hormone that stimulates hepatic glucose production; blocking it may have therapeutic potential in T2DM.

##### Inflammatory Adipokines

Adipose tissue also secretes pro-inflammatory mediators, linking obesity to insulin resistance:

- TNF-α inhibits adipocyte proliferation and differentiation and impairs insulin action by downregulating PPAR-γ.
- IL-6 contributes to obesity-related insulin resistance and suppresses lipoprotein lipase activity.
- Chemokines act as potent chemoattractants and modulators of oxidative and cytokine pathways, promoting chronic low-grade inflammation.

Dysregulated adipokine secretion in obesity serves as a mechanistic link between excess adipose depot, chronic inflammation, insulin resistance, and type 2 diabetes mellitus [6]. Together, the role of leptin and other adipokines along with the lipostat concept highlights adipose tissue role as an endocrine organ.

### 7.2.2 Adipose Tissue Signaling

#### 7.2.2.1 Role of Leptin

Leptin serves as a signal for the status of adipose tissue stores, conveying information to the central nervous system (CNS), mainly hypothalamus [1]. White adipose tissue is the principle source of leptin; however, other sources include the placenta and ovaries, skeletal muscle, and bone marrow. Leptin secretion is directly proportional to adipose tissue depot, where production is seen to increase with increased fat accumulation and decrease with fat loss, thus acting as a physiological indicator of energy reserves in the body [9].

In the hypothalamic neurons of the arcuate nucleus, leptin acts by decreasing the expression of neuropeptide Y (NPY) and agouti-related protein (AgRP). Since NPY is orexigenic and promotes food intake, leptin-mediated inhibition produces an anorexigenic effect. Concurrently, leptin also stimulates the hypothalamic pro-opiomelanocortin (POMC) neurons to increase the synthesis of α-melanocyte-stimulating hormone (α-MSH), further suppressing appetite. Together, these actions decrease hunger and promote weight loss, as suggested by the name of the hormone itself.

An interesting observation in overweight and obese individuals is that leptin levels remain chronically elevated (hyperleptinemia), yet its central effects stay diminished, termed as *leptin resistance*. This results in blunting of the appetite suppressing effect of leptin and leads to the persistence of obesity [5, 9–11].

#### 7.2.2.2 Role of Adiponectin

Adipocytes also produce the hormone adiponectin. While the majority of the adiponectin is derived from adipose cells, another significant source is the placenta. It is also locally expressed in several tissues and acts like an autocrine and paracrine agent. The blood levels of adiponectin are significantly reduced in states of obesity, insulin resistance, and type 2 diabetes mellitus. This demonstrates the close association of adiponectin with metabolic dysfunction. On the contrary,

**Table 7.1** Effects of leptin

| Target | Action(s) | Effect |
|---|---|---|
| Hypothalamus | Inhibits neuropeptide Y and agouti-related protein neurons<br>Stimulates α-melanocyte-stimulating hormone<br>Reverses starvation-induced inhibition of the hypothalamic–pituitary–gonadal and hypothalamic–pituitary–thyroid axes (indirect effect)<br>Stimulates gonadotropin-releasing hormone<br>Causes parasympathetic-induced increased hepatic insulin sensitivity with inhibition of glucose production (arcuate nucleus projections to the nucleus of tractus solitarius) | Anorexigenic effect<br>Hypoglycemic effect<br>Reproductive effect |
| Skeletal muscle | Increases glucose uptake<br>Increases glucose and fatty acid oxidation | Catabolic effect |
| Liver | Decreases gluconeogenesis | Hypoglycemic effect |
| Adipocyte (autocrine activity) | Promotes glucose and fatty acid oxidation<br>Promotes lipolysis<br>Decreases leptin gene expression | Catabolic effect |
| Pancreatic Islets | Inhibits insulin release<br>Decreases glucagon release | Glucoregulatory effect (adipoinsular axis) |
| Adrenal cortex | Decreases adrenocorticotropic hormone-stimulated glucocorticoid release | Decreased insulin antagonism<br>Catabolic effect |
| Immune system cells (permissive effect) | Enhances phagocytic activity of macrophages<br>Stimulates cytokine and chemotaxin production | Immunoprotective effect |
| Bone (permissive) | Increases bone mineral density<br>Increases hematopoiesis | Anabolic skeletal effect |

calorie restriction leads to an increase in the adiponectin concentrations despite a reduction in adipose tissue mass. This demonstrates its role in insulin sensitivity and metabolic homeostasis [1].

Two receptors—AdipoR1 present in skeletal muscles and AdipoR2 present in the liver—mediate the action of adiponectin. Adiponectin increases fatty acid oxidation and insulin sensitivity via the AMPK and PPAR-α signaling pathways. This leads to a decrease in the blood glucose levels, reduced hepatic gluconeogenesis, increased glucose uptake, and increased clearance of triglycerides.

Table 7.1 summarizes the various effects of leptin on its target tissues.

#### 7.2.2.3 Leptin–Adiponectin Ratio (LAR)

An increase in adipose tissue mass results in a rise in leptin levels, hyperleptinemia, and decline in adiponectin levels, hypoadiponectinemia. Both of these phenomena are characteristic features of obesity. Hence, these two hormones serve as markers for metabolic health, reflecting the functional state of adipose tissue. In metabolically healthy individuals with normal adipose tissue mass, the ratio of leptin to adiponectin (leptin–adiponectin ratio) is less than one. In overweight and obese individual, there is increased adipose tissue accumulation, resulting in increase in the LAR ratio to one or more than one [1, 2].

An LAR of one or more is indicative of not just progressive adiposopathy but also vascular stiffness and reduced compliance. It can be used as a reliable indicator for risk of development of metabolic syndrome and vascular disease.

## 7.3 Protein Metabolism

Dietary proteins undergo enzymatic breakdown starting from the stomach, where gastric pepsin cleaves them into smaller fragments, and further breakdown in the duodenum through the action of pancreatic enzymes, trypsin, and chymotrypsin, leading to formation of shorter polypeptides. These intermediate peptides are subsequently degraded by exopeptidases and dipeptidases in the brush-border of enterocytes, ultimately resulting in free amino acids. The absorbed amino acids are then taken up by various tissues, where they act as the fundamental building blocks for protein synthesis. The newly synthesized proteins are required not only for metabolic regulation, but also for maintenance of cellular integrity and production of components of the extracellular matrix.

Amino acid metabolism primarily occurs in the liver. All excess amino acids are transported to the liver where they undergo deamination. Their carbon moiety is directed into metabolic pathways and via the alanine cycle and gluconeogenesis is converted into glucose. The nitrogen released during deamination is utilized to form urea, which is subsequently eliminated via the kidneys. Amino acid catabolism can also generate keto acids. They act as precursors for acetyl-CoA which is a substrate for lipogenesis and subsequent fat storage.

Beyond their role in energy provision, amino acids also influence endocrine and metabolic responses of the body. The source of dietary protein and resulting amino acids affect insulin secretion, increase in adipocyte mass, circulating levels of free fatty acids, and the risk of lipid accumulation in the liver and skeletal muscles [1].

## 7.4 Glucose Metabolism

### 7.4.1 Glucokinase [1]

The hormone glucokinase, belonging to the hexokinase family, plays a central role in carbohydrate metabolism. It acts like a catalyst for the phosphorylation of glucose to glucose-6-phosphate (G6P). This step represents the first, most essential step for both glycolysis and glycogen synthesis. Compared to most other enzymes of the body which have a broad tissue distribution, glucokinase expression is present in four specific mammalian cells only. These are *hepatocytes*, *β-cells* of the pancreas, *enterocytes*, and glucose-sensitive *neurons*. Glucokinase acts like a glucose sensor in these cells and adjusts metabolic and cellular activity in response to fluctuations in glucose levels in plasma. Mutations in the glucokinase gene can lead to disruption of its regulatory function. The affected individuals present with symptoms of monogenic forms of diabetes or, conversely, episodes of hypoglycemia.

Glucokinase differs from the other isoforms of the hexokinase family. It exhibits unique kinetic characteristics, which results in its affinity for glucose to be considerably lower than that of the other isoforms. Glucokinase activity increases proportionally with increase in the blood glucose levels, making it a reliable sensor for postprandial glucose surge. Since it is restricted to four types of localized tissues only, glucose phosphorylation via glucokinase is strictly controlled based on the physiological requirements.

After nutrient ingestion, dietary carbohydrates are initially degraded by salivary and pancreatic amylases to give oligosaccharides. These are further hydrolyzed by disaccharidases present in the brush-border of enterocytes, to produce monosaccharides. Monosaccharides such as glucose, fructose (from sucrose), and galactose (from lactose) are absorbable. Upon absorption, glucose enters the portal circulation and transported directly into the liver, which is the primary organ for postprandial glucose handling and metabolism.

Any subsequent increase in plasma glucose levels leads to stimulation of β-cells of the pancreas to secrete insulin. Under the influence of glucokinase, hepatocytes promote glycogenesis, to store glucose in the form of glycogen. Hence, glucokinase serves as both a metabolic gatekeeper and a sensor, to ensure efficient utilization and storage of dietary glucose.

### 7.4.2 Insulin

Islets of Langerhans in the pancreas are organized in a way that closely links their arrangement to their endocrine function. The arterial blood flow through the pancreatic islets plays a critical role in maintaining the balance between insulin and glucagon secretion from the endocrine pancreas. Blood enters the pancreatic islets in such a pattern that it first perfuses the β-cells located centrally, which in turn secrete insulin. Post this, the blood reaches the α-cells situated peripherally in the islets, which in turn release glucagon. This arrangement also allows insulin to exert a local paracrine influence on glucagon release.

#### 7.4.2.1 Glucose Sensing in β-Cells

The primary glucose sensor expressed by β-cells is glucose transporter 2 (GLUT2). Activation of GLUT2 results in facilitated diffusion of glucose into the cell directly in proportion to the extracellular glucose concentration. Unlike GLUT4, which is the insulin-dependent glucose transporter expressed in adipose tissue and skeletal muscle, GLUT2 is constitutively present in the membrane of the β-cells of pancreas and operates independent of insulin signal. GLUT2 also has a low affinity for glucose. This ensured that significant glucose transport occurs only when the circulating glucose levels are high.

Glucose undergoes phosphorylation by glucokinase inside the cell. Since glucokinase has a relatively low affinity for glucose and is not subject to feedback inhibition by glucose-6-phosphate, it acts most effectively during postprandial glucose surges, maintaining the glycolytic flux in the β-cell.

#### 7.4.2.2 Mechanism of Insulin Secretion

Metabolism of glucose within the β-cells of the pancreas results in an increase in the intracellular adenosine-tri-phosphate (ATP) to adenosine-di-phosphate (ADP) ratio. Intracellular rise in the ATP causes closure of ATP-sensitive potassium (KATP) channels, resulting in membrane depolarization. Depolarization causes opening of voltage-gated calcium channels and movement of calcium into the cell. Increased concentration of intracellular calcium triggers the exocytosis of secretory granules containing insulin, present in its precursor form. During the process of exocytosis, proinsulin is first cleaved, and insulin is subsequently released into the circulation in equimolar amounts with C-peptide [1].

#### 7.4.2.3 Other Endocrine Cell Types in the Islets

In addition to β- and α-cells, the pancreatic islets contain several other hormone-secreting cells: δ-Cells secrete the hormone *somatostatin*, which inhibits both insulin and glucagon release. F-Cells release *pancreatic polypeptide*, which decreases gastric secretion, delays gastric emptying and increasing gastric emptying time, suppresses pancreatic exocrine secretion, decreases biliary secretion, and reduces appetite. ε-Cells produce ghrelin, a hormone primarily derived from the stomach, which inhibits insulin secretion.

#### 7.4.2.4 Nutrient and Hormonal Modulation of Insulin Release

Insulin secretion is not solely driven by glucose. Amino acids stimulate insulin release, particularly when ingested as a mixture, enhancing the β-cell response compared with single amino acid intake. Free fatty acids (FFAs) also augment glucose-stimulated insulin secretion in the fed state. However, chronic elevations in FFA, as seen in obesity and adiposopathy, impair β-cell responsiveness and contribute to insulin resistance.

Gut-derived peptides play an essential role in postprandial insulin secretion. Intestinal L-cells secrete Glucagon-like peptide-1 (GLP-1), whereas enteroendocrine K-cells secrete glucose-dependent insulinotropic polypeptide (GIP). Both GLP-1 and GIP enhance insulin release in response to nutrient ingestion. Impairments in incretin secretion or signaling contribute to defective insulin release and hyperglycemia in metabolic syndrome, obesity and type 2 diabetes mellitus.

#### 7.4.2.5 Inhibition of Insulin Release

Insulin secretion is also subject to inhibitory regulation. In addition to somatostatin and ghrelin, catecholamines act via α2-adrenergic receptors on β-cells to strongly suppress insulin release. This adrenergic inhibition, mediated by adrenaline and norepinephrine, is a key defense mechanism against hypoglycemia. The reduction in insulin, combined with the hyperadrenergic symptoms (sweating, palpitations, and tremors), promotes food-seeking behavior during hypoglycemic episodes.

#### 7.4.2.6 Insulin and Glucagon Dynamics in the Fed and Fasting States

##### Fed State

Following a meal, nutrient-rich blood with elevated glucose content enters the pancreatic islets. The initial exposure of β-cells to this glucose surge stimulates insulin secretion, resulting in high local insulin concentrations. As blood flows downstream to the α-cells, insulin acts in a paracrine manner to suppress glucagon release. The venous outflow from pancreas in the postprandial period is typically characterized by high blood glucose levels and a high insulin-to-glucagon ratio.

This venous blood then enters the portal circulation and reaches the liver, which is the first major target organ. Within the hepatocytes, insulin binds to its receptors and activates pathways for glycogen synthesis (glycogenesis) while simultaneously suppressing pathways for glucose production via gluconeogenesis.

A small amount of the insulin bypasses the liver and enters the systemic circulation, where it exerts metabolic effects on peripheral tissues. In the skeletal muscles, insulin facilitates the translocation of GLUT4 transporters to the plasma membrane to increase glucose uptake and promote glycogen storage. In the adipose tissues, insulin stimulates GLUT4 recruitment to enable glucose entry into the cell to provide glycerol for triglyceride synthesis. Insulin also activates lipoprotein lipase on the adipocyte surface, to hydrolyze circulating triglycerides into free fatty acids, which are then esterified and stored. Insulin also suppresses hormone-sensitive lipases to prevent lipolysis. The overall action of insulin on adipose tissue is mainly lipogenic to promote the retention of fatty acids within the fat depots.

##### Fasting State

During fasting states, blood that enters the pancreatic islets has normal (or reduced) levels of glucose. Normal or reduced glucose uptake by the pancreatic β-cells leads to a decline in insulin secretion. As a result, blood reaching the α-cells in the periphery of the islets has low insulin levels, thus removing the inhibitory paracrine influence of insulin on glucagon secretion from α-cells. The pancreatic venous outflow in this state thus contains normal glucose, less insulin, and elevated glucagon levels, that is, low insulin-to-glucagon ratio.

Upon reaching the liver via the portal vein, there is a shift in metabolism. In the absence of insulin, glucagon predominates and causes glycogen breakdown (glycogenolysis) to maintain the plasma glucose levels. With prolonged fasting, glucagon not only causes glycogenolysis but also enhances gluconeogenesis, ensuring a continuous supply of glucose for tissues, particularly the brain and red blood cells, that rely on glucose as their primary source of energy.

#### 7.4.2.7 Insulin Actions in the CNS

Insulin receptors are expressed widely in the central nervous system (CNS). Within the brain, insulin signaling plays a central role in metabolism, regulation of food intake, and maintenance of energy balance. Just like leptin, insulin also functions as an adiposity signal to the hypothalamus, informing the brain about peripheral energy stores.

Insulin is transported into the CNS across the blood–brain barrier via receptor-mediated mechanisms. It then binds to receptors located mainly in hypothalamic nuclei and in some extrahypothalamic regions. The downstream effects of insulin include modulation of appetite, regulation of activity of the sympathetic nervous system, and insulin sensitivity. At the molecular level, both hormones, insulin and leptin, share activation of the phosphatidylinositol 3-kinase (PI3K) pathway. Impairment of this pathway affects insulin action and leads to increased insulin resistance.

Apart from its metabolic effects, insulin also plays a role in neuronal health. One important target is the tau protein, a microtubule-associated protein which stabilizes cytoskeletal structure. In conditions of impaired insulin activity or increased insulin resistance, tau undergoes abnormal phosphorylation. This leads to the formation of paired helical filaments and neurofibrillary tangles. These aggregates serve as a neuropathological hallmark of Alzheimer's disease, and their presence correlates with the severity of cognitive decline, linking insulin resistance with neurodegenerative processes.

Insulin also plays an important role in regulation of amyloid precursor protein to facilitate the clearance of β-amyloid from the brain. Reduced insulin activity

**Table 7.2** Effects of insulin

| Target | Action(s) | Effect |
|---|---|---|
| Adipocytes | Induces lipoprotein lipase activity (influx of FFA into adipocytes)<br>Inhibits hormone-sensitive lipase (stops efflux of FFA)<br>Increases glucose uptake (GLUT4) | Lipogenesis |
| Hepatocytes | Inhibits glycogenolysis and gluconeogenesis<br>Inhibits conversion of fatty acids and amino acids to keto acids<br>Promotes glycogenesis (inhibits phosphorylase; stimulates glucokinase, and glycogen synthase)<br>Increases triglyceride synthesis and very low-density lipoprotein formation | Glycogenesis |
| Brain | Causes satiety<br>Increases energy expenditure | Anorexigenic effect |
| Muscle | Increases amino acid transport and protein synthesis<br>Increases glucose uptake (GLUT4) and glycogen synthase activity<br>Inhibits phosphorylase | Glycogenesis<br>Anabolic effect |
| Pancreas | Inhibits glucagon release | Hypoglycemic effect |

*FFA* free fatty acids, *GLUT* glucose transporter

leads to β-amyloid accumulation, further linking insulin resistance with neurodegenerative processes. Insulin signaling, via various mechanisms, thus represents a critical link between energy homeostasis, neuroprotection, and cognitive health. Table 7.2 summarizes the various actions and effects of insulin on its target tissues.

The endocrine regulation of metabolism is central not only to the maintenance of normal energy balance but also to the pathogenesis of metabolic disease. Type 2 diabetes mellitus (T2DM) represents a prime example for endocrine and metabolic dysregulation. Diabetes mellitus results from pancreatic β-cell dysfunction and increased insulin resistance in peripheral tissues, leading to relative insulin deficiency, high plasma glucose, and associated symptoms.

Initially, the underlying pathophysiology of diabetes was conceptualized [6] as the "triumvirate" [27], which included defects in three organs involved in glucose homeostasis: the pancreas (impaired insulin secretion), skeletal muscle (increased insulin resistance), and the liver (increased hepatic glucose production). Later, this view was broadened into the "ominous octet" (DeFronzo 2009), incorporating the contributions of adipose tissue (accelerated lipolysis), incretin hormones (defective secretion and action), α-cells (hyperglucagonemia), the kidney (enhanced glucose reabsorption), and the brain (neurotransmitter dysfunction and appetite dysregulation) in the pathophysiology of diabetes.

Kalra et al. [28] added the role of dopamine, vitamin D, testosterone, and the renin–angiotensin system, and proposed the "dirty dozen", while Somasundaram and Wijesinghe [26, 29] included the roles of the gut and gut microbiota, iron overload, and gut-derived serotonin in the development of diabetes, calling them the "unlucky thirteen". Collectively, these models suggest that diabetes mellitus is not just the result of dysfunction in a single pathway but also a multisystem disorder, closely linked to hormonal networks that govern energy balance under normal physiological conditions [12].

Since regulation of energy balance is primarily dependent on pancreatic β-cell function and insulin action, any disruption whether by insulin resistance (as in type 2 diabetes mellitus) or by autoimmune β-cell destruction (as in type 1 diabetes mellitus) leads to disturbances in glucose metabolism and overall energy homeostasis.

Type 1 diabetes mellitus (T1DM) is an autoimmune disease characterized by progressive loss of pancreatic β-cells ultimately leading to absolute insulin deficiency. The natural history of type 1 diabetes has been classically described by the Eisenbarth model [6], which outlines a stepwise progression:

Stage I—Stage of genetic susceptibility: It is characterized by the presence of specific HLA haplotypes and other risk alleles that make the individual vulnerable to β-cell autoimmunity.

Stage II—Stage of environmental trigger/insult: The presence of external factors such as viral infections, dietary influences, etcetera initiates the autoimmune cascade in genetically susceptible individuals.

Stage III—Stage of active autoimmunity: It is associated with the emergence of islet-directed autoantibodies. The presence of these antibodies reflects ongoing immune-mediated injury, although glucose tolerance remains intact.

Stage IV—Stage of metabolic abnormalities: It is associated with progressive β-cell loss. It leads to subclinical defects in glucose homeostasis and presents with impaired glucose tolerance on investigation.

Stage V—Stage of clinical diabetes: Once β-cell number and function falls below a critical threshold, overt hyperglycemia and the classical symptoms of diabetes manifest.

Stage VI—Stage of insulin dependence: Near-total or total β-cell destruction resulting in use of exogenous insulin for survival and metabolic regulation

Hence "triumvirate," "ominous octet," and "dirty dozen" highlight the multisystem pathophysiology of type 2 diabetes; the "Eisenbarth" stages of T1DM underscore the central role of β-cell number and function in maintaining metabolic balance.

Although both the types of diabetes mellitus arise from distinct mechanisms, they ultimately reflect a failure of the endocrine system to maintain energy homeostasis. In T1DM, the absence of insulin affects the ability to regulate glucose uptake and utilization, whereas in T2DM, insulin is present but ineffective due to peripheral resistance. Together, these disorders highlight pathways through which the finely tuned hormonal control of metabolism can break down: one through absolute deficiency and the other through relative insufficiency and resistance.

## 7.5 Gut Hormones

The role of the intestine apart from digestion of nutrients and the absorption of food components is also a key regulator of metabolism through its neural and hormonal outputs. At the time of digestion, the arrival of nutrients in the gastrointestinal tract initiates a series of events. Gut-derived signals are transmitted through the enteric nervous system and by the release of hormones from specialized enteroendocrine cells. These signals then provide feedback to the central nervous system, to regulate appetite and satiety. Gut hormones also coordinate with peripheral organs, such as the pancreas, liver, and adipose tissue, to control handling of nutrients and utilization of energy.

### 7.5.1 Ghrelin

After the ingested food reaches the stomach, the mechanical breakdown of food due to muscular contractions, secretion of hydrochloric acid, and the release of digestive enzymes that initiate protein digestion in the stomach begins. Apart from digestion, the stomach also regulates energy balance via signaling pathways with the central nervous system. This bidirectional signaling is mediated mainly by vagal afferents and efferents, involving neural control of gastric function, as well as the feedback from the stomach to the brain.

In addition to the neural pathways, several hormones help in stomach and brain communication. These hormones include:

- Nesfatin, a peptide expressed in the hypothalamus, endocrine cells of the stomach, pancreatic islets, and adipose tissue
- Signaling molecules of the gastric endocannabinoid system; and
- Ghrelin, secreted primarily by the stomach

The identification of ghrelin was closely linked to the research involving mediators of growth hormone release. In 1996, a G protein-coupled receptor was discovered in the pituitary and the arcuate, ventromedial, and infundibular nuclei of the hypothalamus. This receptor was initially recognized as the target for synthetic growth hormone secretagogues. Eventually, in 1999, its endogenous ligand was isolated and named ghrelin, due to its role in growth hormone secretion.

Ghrelin is primarily secreted by a group of endocrine cells known as X/A-like cells (or P/D1 cells) which are present in the mucosa of oxyntic cells of the stomach. Epsilon cells of the pancreas and certain neuronal populations in the hypothalamus also secrete ghrelin in minute quantities. The pattern of secretion dependent on the nutrient status of the individual, circulating levels of ghrelin increase during fasting states, peaks just before food intake and drops rapidly once feeding begins. Distension of the stomach leads to suppression of ghrelin secretion. The maximum postprandial decline occurs after the ingestion of protein or carbohydrate, as compared to fat which has a weak inhibitory effect.

Ghrelin is encoded by the GHRL gene in the form of a large inactive precursor. The precursor yields preproghrelin, a 117-amino acid peptide which is structurally similar to promotilin. Preproghrelin breaks down to give proghrelin, which undergoes further cleavage to generate the unacylated 28-amino acid ghrelin peptide. Further processing produces c-ghrelin, an acylated variant, and then obestatin, which is opposes ghrelin's physiological actions.

Ghrelin undergoes post-translational modification to become biologically active. The enzyme ghrelin O-acyltransferase (GOAT), located on the membrane of gastric Gr cells, attaches an octanoic acid moiety to the third-position serine residue on ghrelin. It is the acylated form of ghrelin that is capable of binding and activating the growth hormone secretagogue receptor (GHSR). The unacylated form of ghrelin lacks receptor activity, and its functions in terms of modulating appetite and glucose metabolism are the opposite of acylated ghrelin.

#### 7.5.1.1 Regulation of Ghrelin and Energy Balance

Ghrelin acts as a signal for negative energy balance. It helps promote hunger and stimulate food intake. Its levels in the blood vary with nutritional and pathological status. For instance, obesity is generally associated with reduced circulating ghrelin concentrations compared to lean individuals; in Prader–Willi syndrome, ghrelin remains chronically elevated and results in hyperphagia

**Table 7.3** Effects of ghrelin

| Target | Action(s) | Effect |
|---|---|---|
| Stomach | Increases gastric acid secretion<br>Increases gastric motility<br>Decreases the mechanosensitivity of gastric vagal afferent nerves (makes them less sensitive to gastric distention) | Prepares the stomach for food intake |
| Intestine | Promotes intestinal cell proliferation<br>Inhibits intestinal cell apoptosis during inflammation<br>Suppresses pro-inflammatory mechanisms<br>Augments anti-inflammatory mechanisms<br>Stimulates regeneration of gastric mucosa | Intestinal healing and anti-inflammatory effect |
| Pancreatic islets of Langerhans | Inhibits glucose-stimulated insulin secretion by β-cells (indirect effect)<br>Stimulates somatostatin release by δ-cells (direct effect) | Hypoglycemic effect |
| Hippocampus | Regulates neurotrophy<br>Alters neuronal connections | Stimulates learning and memory |
| Pituitary | Stimulates growth hormone release<br>Stimulates ACTH release | Stimulates growth and development<br>Antidepressant effect<br>Anxiolytic effect |
| Hypothalamic arcuate nucleus | Stimulates orexigenic neuropeptide Y and agouti-related protein neurons<br>Increases hunger<br>Inhibits gonadotropin-releasing hormone | Orexigenic effect<br>Increase body weight and fat mass<br>Decreases fertility |
| Dopamine neurons that link ventral tegmental area to nucleus accumbens | Produces sensations of reward and reinforcement<br>Contributes to the development of addictions | Hedonism regarding foods and drugs like alcohol |
| Endothelium | Activates nitric oxide synthase | Vasodilator |
| Lung | Promotes lung growth early in fetal life | Lung growth |

which is commonly seen in this syndrome; in disorders of energy deficiency, such as anorexia nervosa and cancer-associated cachexia, ghrelin concentrations are highly elevated to increase calorie intake; and aging is accompanied by gradual elevations in circulating ghrelin. This gradual increase leads to fat accumulation later in life.

Therapeutic interventions such as bariatric surgery, including Roux-en-Y gastric bypass and sleeve gastrectomy, significantly reduce circulating ghrelin and disrupt its normal pre- and post-meal fluctuations in the blood. This suppression in circulating ghrelin contributes toward a reduced appetite and sustained weight loss after surgery.

In the CNS, ghrelin receptors are located on neuronal cells that also express leptin and insulin receptors, suggesting its role in linking adiposity and nutrient signals. Ghrelin acts as an orexigenic neuropeptide to stimulate food intake. In doing so, it opposes leptin's anorexigenic effects and complements the role of insulin. In the peripheral tissues, ghrelin helps direct energy toward ATP production or storage, either in the form of triglycerides in adipose tissue or as glycogen in the liver. It also causes short-term heat loss, energy expenditure, and utilization. These effects have been summarized in Table 7.3.

Thus, along with leptin and insulin, ghrelin also contributes toward coordination of the neuroendocrine system to integrate central and peripheral signals to maintain energy homeostasis. Disruption of this balance leads to the development of not only metabolic disorders such as obesity and insulin resistance but also cachexia. Therapeutically, ghrelin agonists and analogs are being explored for anorexia nervosa and cancer cachexia, while antagonism of ghrelin signaling may hold potential in the treatment of obesity.

### 7.5.2 Obestatin

Obestatin was discovered in 2005 as a peptide product derived from the same GHRL gene that encodes ghrelin. It is generated through post-translational cleavage of c-ghrelin, and its principal site of production is the stomach. Additional expression has been documented in multiple tissues, including the duodenum, jejunum, colon, pancreas, thyroid, lungs, mammary glands, spleen, skeletal muscle, adipose tissue, and in the Leydig cells of the testes. For obestatin to attain biological activity, the C-terminal glycine residue must undergo amidation, a modification essential for receptor interaction. The specific enzyme catalyzing this amidation remains unidentified.

Specific binding sites for obestatin have been reported in the pancreas, heart, and white adipose tissue. Although a specific obestatin receptor has not been identified, evidence suggests obestatin possibly interacts with GLP-1 receptor expressed by pancreatic β-cells and adipocytes.

In the pancreatic ε-cells, obestatin is co-expressed along with ghrelin. This co-expression suggests that ghrelin and obestatin act together and regulate β-cell activity. However, obestatin is not co-expressed with any other pancreatic hormone insulin, glucagon, or somatostatin. Hence, ghrelin also acts within the pancreas through autocrine and paracrine mechanisms, apart from similar systemic effects.

In the adipose tissues, obestatin promotes cell growth and proliferation by regulating gene expression. It also helps in adipocyte differentiation and adipose tissue remodeling. It has been shown to play a protective role in cytokine-induced apoptosis and during inflammatory stress.

In humans, circulating levels of obestatin remain relatively stable after fixed and low calorie meals, showing only minimal fluctuation with controlled, short-term nutrient intake. Obese individuals typically have lower plasma levels of obestatin in comparison with lean individuals. This observation is suggestive of their potential role in the long-term regulation of adiposity and stored fat mass. An elevated ghrelin-to-obestatin ratio, particularly in the fasting state, has been reported in individuals with obesity. Such dysregulation may represent a mechanistic factor in the progression of overweight and obesity, as well as in adipose tissue pathology.

### 7.5.3 Proglucagon and GLP-1

The proglucagon gene is expressed in pancreatic α-cells, enteroendocrine L-cells, and specific neuronal populations in the brainstem and hypothalamus. Although the same gene is expressed in all these cell populations, the peptides derived from them differ and are tissue-specific. In the pancreas, α-cells primarily produce glucagon, whereas in the intestine and central nervous system, they produce glicentin, glucagon-like peptide-1 (GLP-1), and glucagon-like peptide-2 (GLP-2). Cleavage of glicentin results in production of glicentin-related pancreatic peptide (GRPP) and oxyntomodulin.

GLP-1, released mainly from intestinal L-cells and neurons of the nucleus tractus solitarius, is a 30-amino acid peptide. Its secretion is stimulated by nutrient ingestion. The initial, non-active translation product, GLP-1(1–37), undergoes amidation and proteolysis, to produce two biologically active isoforms: GLP-1(7–36) and GLP-1(7–37). Both act as potent incretin hormones, to enhance insulin secretion in response to glucose stimulation.

Beyond regulation of glucose, GLP-1 also exerts actions on the central nervous system by reducing the meal size and frequency, decreasing reward-driven food consumption, lowering the locomotor activity, and enhancing hippocampal processes such as learning and memory. GLP-1 signaling also promotes the formation of conditioned taste aversions and can induce nausea, anxiety, and visceral discomfort, effects relevant both physiologically and pharmacologically.

At the level of the pancreas, GLP-1 enhances β-cell proliferation, increases insulin biosynthesis and secretion, and augments α- and β-cell insulin sensitivity. It also suppresses glucagon release through its action on to GLP-1 receptors present on the α-cells. In the gastrointestinal tract, GLP-1 acts by reducing the secretion of gastric acid and increasing gastric emptying time to help control postprandial glucose spikes.

In the peripheral tissues, GLP-1 increases insulin sensitivity and promotes glucose utilization. However, endogenous GLP-1 is rapidly inactivated by enzymes dipeptidyl peptidase-4 (DPP-4) and neutral endopeptidase, and it has a very short half-life of ~2 min. Hence, only about 10–15% of the secreted GLP-1 enters systemic circulation in active form, while the remaining inactivated GLP-1 is cleared, primarily by the kidneys.

GLP-1 also contributes toward adipose tissue regulation. The active form of GLP-1 facilitates adipogenesis by promoting preadipocyte proliferation and protecting against apoptosis. Conversely, loss of GLP-1 receptor signaling reduces adipocyte development and enhances apoptosis. GLP-1(9–36), which is a DPP-4 generated metabolite, lacks affinity for GLP-1 receptor and inhibits cell proliferation, glucose uptake, and adipogenesis in human adipose stem cells while promoting apoptosis. GLP-1 is not just an incretin hormone that helps regulate insulin secretion and postprandial glucose metabolism but also helps modulate appetite, gastrointestinal, and islet cell function, along with adipose tissue regulation [12–16].

## 7.6 Other Endocrine Influences on Metabolism

Metabolic regulation is not only restricted to pancreatic hormones alone but is also shaped by signals originating from the hypothalamus–pituitary axis. Among these, thyroid hormones play a particularly significant role in coordinating energy turnover and tissue responsiveness.

### 7.6.1 Thyroid Hormones: Triiodothyronine and Thyroxine

The thyroid gland, through its follicular cells, synthesizes two closely related hormones: thyroxine (tetraiodothyronine, T4) and triiodothyronine (T3). In the circulation, T4 is the major secretory product and exists in much higher concentrations than T3, with a plasma T4:T3 ratio typically ranging between 14:1 and 20:1. Despite being present in larger quantities, T4 serves largely as a prohormone. Peripheral tissues and thyroid gland convert the less active T4 into more active T3 with the help of deiodinase (5′-iodinase) enzymes. T3 is the more biologically potent form. It exhibits nearly five times greater activity than T4 and is therefore considered the principal effector hormone.

Thyroid hormone receptors, particularly T3 receptors, are expressed in nearly all body tissues. It exerts a wide range of actions on metabolism and development via these receptors. One function of importance is the elevation of basal metabolic rate, which is brought about by enhancing the tissue sensitivity to circulating catecholamines. Other functions include, but are not limited to, growth, cellular differentiation, and functional maturation of organs.

T3 acts by increasing the heart rate and thereby the cardiac output. It also increases the respiratory drive and sympathetic activity. T3 leads to protein and carbohydrate catabolism. It acts on the gastrointestinal tract to reduce the transit time. In the skeletal muscle, T3 is responsible for increase in contractility. In the adipose tissue, T3 regulates differentiation of adipocytes via reactivation of brown adipose tissue and formation of beige ("brite") adipocytes, which help in non-shivering thermogenesis and energy expenditure during adaption.

Thyroid hormones are closely linked to endocrine regulators of metabolism. Catecholamines and thyroid hormones act synergistically. T3 amplifies the adrenergic signals to increase energy utilization. Insulin provides a counterbalance to thyroid hormones by promoting anabolic processes such as glycogen and lipid synthesis. In adipose tissue, the interplay between thyroid hormones and insulin determines the balance between lipogenesis and lipolysis. In overweight and obese states, the reduced expression of thyroid-regulated genes in subcutaneous and visceral fat depots results in reduced thyroid hormone signaling. Conversely, in lean individuals and during significant weight loss, there is restoration of thyroid-related gene activity, resulting in increased hormone sensitivity.

## 7.6.2 Adrenal Hormones

The adrenal gland secretes two major groups of hormones: steroids secreted mainly from the adrenal cortex and catecholamines secreted from the adrenal medulla. Both these classes of hormones play an important role in metabolism. The actions of both steroids and catecholamines are opposite to that of insulin, particularly in the adipose tissues. While insulin promotes fat storage through lipogenesis, adrenal hormones favor fat mobilization and lipolysis.

### 7.6.2.1 Glucocorticoids

Cortisol is secreted by the zona fasciculata of the adrenal cortex and is the principal glucocorticoid in humans. It has a wide range of metabolic actions including immune regulation and development, but its most prominent metabolic action is the maintenance of energy balance under conditions of stress or fasting. It acts primarily as a catabolic hormone and helps mobilize stored substrates to ensure adequate fuel supply to all the tissues, especially during stress when exogenous nutrients are scarce.

Cortisol stimulates hormone-sensitive lipase, resulting in lipolysis of adipose tissue stores to release fatty acids into the circulation. It acts as an antagonist of insulin on adipocytes and myocytes, to reduce glucose uptake and promote substrate mobilization rather than storage. It also suppresses adiponectin secretion from white adipose tissue, resulting in reduced insulin sensitivity.

In the liver, cortisol causes gluconeogenesis by upregulating key enzymes involved in glucose synthesis. It also mobilizes amino acids to the liver from extrahepatic sites to serve as substrates. Cortisol thus plays a role in shifting metabolism away from the anabolic state of energy storage toward a catabolic state of energy mobilization.

Adipose tissue-derived signals have an influence on adrenal function, establishing a reciprocal relationship between energy homeostasis and stress regulation. Adrenocortical cells also express leptin receptors. Through the action of these receptors, leptin acts by suppressing corticotropin-induced steroidogenesis. Leptin acts not only directly on the adrenals but also at higher levels of the hypothalamic–pituitary–adrenal (HPA) axis. Leptin deficiency has been shown to increase HPA axis activity, suggesting that leptin normally decreases HPA function. Apart from leptin, adiponectin receptors also are present throughout the adrenal cortex and medulla and modulate adrenal output. Adiponectin downregulates steroidogenic enzymes to decrease corticosterone and aldosterone production.

The adipose–adrenal cortex interaction closely integrates metabolic and stress responses, with cortisol as a critical mediator of anabolic and catabolic states of the body in response to environmental influences.

#### 7.6.2.2 Epinephrine

The adrenal medulla can be considered to function as an extension of the sympathetic nervous system. It secretes catecholamines, with epinephrine (adrenaline) being the prominent hormone. Epinephrine acts via adrenergic receptors widely distributed across all the tissues. However, the physiological response depends not only on the adrenergic receptor subtype but also on the location of the target cell. The key metabolic actions of epinephrine include but are not limited to suppression of insulin release from β-cells of the pancreas through α-adrenergic receptors, glycogen breakdown in liver and skeletal muscles, mediated by α-receptors, stimulation of glycolysis in skeletal muscles, inhibition of insulin dependent glycogen synthesis in muscles, increased glucagon secretion from α-cells of pancreas via β-adrenergic receptor activation, and stimulation of adrenocorticotropic hormone (ACTH) release from the anterior pituitary via β-adrenergic receptors.

Epinephrine binds to β-adrenergic receptor, first described in adipocytes, to activate hormone-sensitive lipase causing lipolysis in adipose tissues.

Adipose tissue and the adrenal medulla also interact with each other reciprocally. Leptin stimulates release of catecholamines via leptin receptors present in the adrenal medulla, whereas resistin inhibits catecholamine release. In turn, catecholamines regulate adipose tissue function by increasing pro-inflammatory cytokine production and reduction in leptin and resistin secretion. This bidirectional adipose–adrenal medulla interaction also forms an important component of neuroendocrine and metabolic integration.

## 7.7 Applied Aspects: Correlating Hypotheses with Endocrine Regulation of Metabolism

The endocrine regulation of metabolism is not only essential for maintaining energy homeostasis but also provides an understanding as to how and why disturbances in genes, early life, and environment predispose individuals to metabolic disorders such as obesity and diabetes. Several hypotheses have been proposed in this regard that try to explain the development of these disorders, highlighting the interplay between hormones, genetic influences, and environmental exposures.

### 7.7.1 Evolutionary Perspectives: The Thrifty Genotype

Neel's thrifty genotype [17] hypothesis (1962) proposed that certain genetic traits favor efficient energy storage and insulin action. Early man was a hunter and gatherer and did not have a steady supply of nutrients. He was exposed to environments resulting in states of feast and famine. Neel proposed that when food was in plenty, any excess nutrient was stored for a time when food would be scarce. To achieve this, man had a thrifty gene, advantageous for efficient fat storage for survival. However, in the modern scenario, there is access to food and its availability leading to nutritional abundance. Genetic traits for efficient energy storage were advantageous in the past but cause obesity and diabetes today. Although important, this hypothesis oversimplified the role of genetics without an explanation about the role of nutrition (and environmental, cultural, and lifestyle factors) in pathogenesis of metabolic disorders.

### 7.7.2 Developmental Origins: Thrifty Phenotype and Fetal Programming

Hales and Barker (1992) proposed the thrifty phenotype [18] hypothesis, which emphasizes that maternal malnutrition and other maternal and placental abnormalities lead to fetal malnutrition. This resulted in reduced β-cell mass and altered islet function. The result was further compromised in fetal growth and eventually abnormal adult β-cell function. In postnatal life, especially when these individuals are exposed to calorie abundance, the insult in utero predisposes the individuals to develop insulin resistance, diabetes, and metabolic syndrome. This hypothesis also forms the basis of fetal programming hypothesis, which suggests that intrauterine exposure to adverse conditions alters long-term, post-natal endocrine regulation of metabolism.

Evidence in view of this can be obtained from the Dutch Famine [19] Birth Cohort (Stein and Susser 1975), where infants exposed to famine during early trimester had higher adult obesity rates, compared to infants exposed during midtrimester. Similarly, the Rochester [20] study (Charney et al. 1976) showed that there is a substantial correlation between weight attained in the first 6 months of life and adult weight status in the third decade of life. These studies reinforced the idea that early endocrine adaptations influence lifelong metabolic control.

### 7.7.3 Adaptive Mechanisms: Fetal Salvage and Catch-Up Growth

Hofman et al. (1997) proposed the fetal salvage [21] hypothesis, whereby malnourished infants with nutrients inadequate for optimal growth leading to intrauterine growth restriction (IUGR) develop peripheral insulin resistance to ensure adequate glucose delivery to essential organs. Increased insulin resistance results in redistribution of nutrient supply within the fetus, ultimately resulting in permanent reduction in insulin-responsive skeletal muscle GLUT number and/or function. The increased insulin resistance also stimulates β-cells to secrete more insulin. These endocrine adaptations predispose the individuals to eventual β-cell exhaustion and development of diabetes later in life.

Cianfarani et al. (1999) introduced the catch-up growth [22] hypothesis, which also discussed infants with IUGR with limited supply of glucose and results in switching of the IGF (insulin like growth factor) system. Adequate postnatal nutrient supply activates IGF system, leading to catch-up growth and insulin resistance. IUGR children show a rearrangement of the endocrine system at birth, with low concentrations of insulin, IGF-I, IGFBP-3, and high concentrations of growth hormone, IGFBP-1,and IGFBP-2. When these parameters are normalized during the first trimester of postnatal life, the tissues that were chronically depleted of insulin and IGF-I during fetal life and suddenly exposed to increased concentrations of the two hormones shortly after birth may counteract their additive insulin-like actions by developing insulin resistance as a metabolic defense mechanism to protect them from hypoglycemia. This ultimately increases their risk of developing obesity and type 2 diabetes mellitus later in life.

### 7.7.4 Epigenetic Perspectives: The Thrifty Epigenotype

To explain and link the heritability of metabolic syndromes and environmental contributions, Stöger (2008) proposed the thrifty epigenotype [23] hypothesis. Stöger suggested that metabolic thrift was an ancient, complex trait which resulted in efficient acquisition, storage and use of energy. He also discussed the presence of an environmentally responsive gene network encoding the trait can undergo genetic canalization. DNA sequence polymorphisms played a minor role in obesity and type 2 diabetes etiology, and disease susceptibility was predominantly determined by epigenetic variations. Leptin gene was the candidate gene for acquisition of a thrifty epigenotype, to exemplify how adipose cell-derived signals link with endocrine control energy balance and play a role in development of metabolic disturbances.

### 7.7.5 Mechanistic Pathways of Fetal Programming

Several endocrine and molecular mechanisms support these hypotheses [24, 25]:

- *Epigenetic programming:* permanent alterations in β-cell mass, adipocyte development, and insulin signaling
- *Glucocorticoid programming:* Excess fetal cortisol exposure alters hypothalamic–pituitary–adrenal axis function and β-cell development.
- *Mitochondrial programming:* impaired mtDNA density and function predispose to insulin resistance
- *Oxidative stress programming:* Intrauterine hypoxia and reactive oxygen species damage β-cells and vascular endothelium.
- *Nutrient sensing pathways (mTOR, OGT):* Dysregulated placental nutrient transfer alters fetal endocrine and metabolic trajectories.

The hypotheses demonstrate that obesity and diabetes, alone or as part of metabolic syndrome, are not just lifestyle disorders but also represent outcomes of a disrupted endocrine regulation of metabolism across the entire life course. Preconception, intrauterine, and postpartum and early life exposure status, in various capacities, can recalibrate and affect insulin secretion, resistance, adipokine

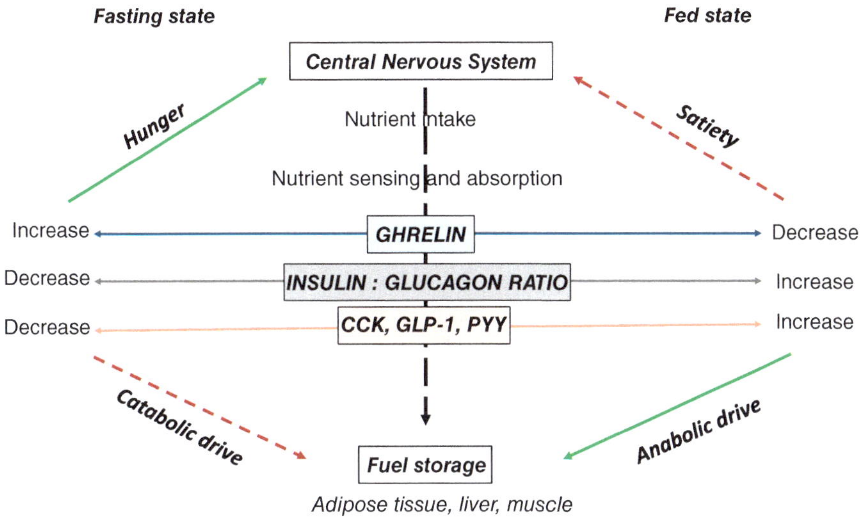


**Fig. 7.2** Signaling pathways for energy balance. Positive or stimulatory influences are represented as solid green arrows, while negative or inhibitory influences are represented as dashed red arrows. After food intake, signals are generated to suppress further feeding and lead to a feeling of satiety. The signals also promote energy storage and are called anabolic drive. As the time after consuming a meal increases, there is a shift in these signals: The feeling of hunger is reinitiated, food intake starts, and energy stores are mobilized; this state is the catabolic drive. *CCK* cholecystokinin, *GLP-1* glucagon-like peptide-1, *PYY* peptide YY

balance, and energy sensing pathways, to increase the risk for T2DM, obesity, hypertension, and cardiovascular disease.

By linking evolutionary, developmental, and molecular hypotheses, we learn that the hormonal regulation of energy metabolism is highly sensitive throughout the life course of an individual. Any mismatch during evolution, development, or at molecular level, results in obesity, diabetes, and other disorders of metabolic health.

## 7.8 Conclusion

Adipose tissue functions as a dynamic regulator of metabolic activity rather than simply a passive energy store. Through its receptors, adipocytes and surrounding cells can sense and respond to signals from other organs involved in nutrient and energy regulation. The nature of this response is determined by the balance between anabolic and catabolic influences (Fig. 7.2). Insulin serves as the principal anabolic hormone, stimulating triglyceride storage within adipocyte lipid droplets. In contrast, catabolic inputs such as adrenaline and cortisol stimulate lipolysis, mobilizing stored fat. Beyond responding to external cues, adipose tissue itself communicates with other organs through endocrine signals. Two of its key hormones are leptin, which informs the central nervous system about energy reserves, and adiponectin, which reflects the functional state of adipose tissue. The relative levels of leptin and adiponectin are now recognized as an important indicator of long-term adipose tissue health.

## References


1. Gonzalez-Campoy JM. Hormonal regulation of energy balance and energy stores. In: Gonzalez-Campoy JM, Hurley DL, Garvey WT, editors. Bariatric endocrinology [Internet]. Cham: Springer International Publishing; 2019 [cited 2025 Aug 31]. p. 37–57. Available from: http://link.springer.com/10.1007/978-3-319-95655-8_3.
2. Suneja M, Murry DJ, Stokes JB, Lim VS. Hormonal regulation of energy-protein homeostasis in hemodialysis patients: an anorexigenic profile that may predispose to adverse cardiovascular outcomes. Am J Physiol-Endocrinol Metab. 2011;300(1):E55–64.
3. Breen DM, Rasmussen BA, Côté CD, Jackson VM, Lam TKT. Nutrient-sensing mechanisms in the gut as therapeutic targets for diabetes. Diabetes. 2013;62(9):3005–13.
4. Müller MJ, Enderle J, Bosy-Westphal A. Changes in energy expenditure with weight gain and weight loss in humans. Curr Obes Rep. 2016;5(4):413–23.
5. Kennedy GC. The role of depot fat in the hypothalamic control of food intake in the rat. Proc R Soc Lond B Biol Sci. 1953;140(901):578–92.
6. Rodriguez-Saldana J, editor. The diabetes textbook: clinical principles, patient management and public health issues [Internet]. Cham: Springer International Publishing; 2023 [cited 2025 Aug 31]. Available from: https://link.springer.com/10.1007/978-3-031-25519-9.
7. Pan WW, Myers MG. Leptin and the maintenance of elevated body weight. Nat Rev Neurosci. 2018;19(2):95–105.
8. Kuo CH, Lai YH, Lin YL, Wang CH, Hsu BG. Fasting serum resistin level positively correlates with metabolic syndrome in patients on peritoneal dialysis. Int J Clin Exp Pathol. 2018 Aug 1;11(8):4257-4263. PMID: 31949821; PMCID: PMC6962780.
9. Fève B, Bastard JP. From the conceptual basis to the discovery of leptin. Biochimie. 2012;94(10):2065–8.
10. Magni P, Motta M, Martini L. Leptin: a possible link between food intake, energy expenditure, and reproductive function. Regul Pept. 2000;92(1–3):51–6.
11. Elmquist JK. Hypothalamic pathways underlying the endocrine, autonomic, and behavioral effects of leptin. Int J Obes Relat Metab Disord. 2001 Dec;25 Suppl 5:S78-82. doi: 10.1038/sj.ijo.0801918. PMID: 11840221.
12. Ralph A DeFronzo; The Triumvirate: β-Cell, Muscle, Liver: A Collusion Responsible for NIDDM. Diabetes 1988;37(6):667–687. https://doi.org/10.2337/diab.37.6.667.
13. Brubaker PL. Minireview: update on incretin biology: focus on glucagon-like peptide-1. Endocrinology. 2010;151(5):1984–9.
14. Sun F, Chai S, Li L, Yu K, Yang Z, Wu S, et al. Effects of glucagon-like peptide-1 receptor agonists on weight loss in patients with type 2 diabetes: a systematic review and network meta-analysis. J Diabetes Res. 2015;2015:1–9.
15. Vilsboll T, Christensen M, Junker AE, Knop FK, Gluud LL. Effects of glucagon-like peptide-1 receptor agonists on weight loss: systematic review and meta-analyses of randomised controlled trials. BMJ. 2012;344(jan10 2):d7771.
16. Cantini G, Di Franco A, Mannucci E, Luconi M. Is cleaved glucagon-like peptide 1 really inactive? Effects of GLP-1(9-36) on human adipose stem cells. Mol Cell Endocrinol. 2017;439:10–5.
17. Abu-Hamdah R, Rabiee A, Meneilly GS, Shannon RP, Andersen DK, Elahi D. The extrapancreatic effects of glucagon-like peptide-1 and related peptides. J Clin Endocrinol Metab. 2009;94(6):1843–52.
18. NEEL JV. Diabetes mellitus: a thrifty genotype rendered detrimental by progress? Am J Hum Genet. 1962 Dec;14(4):353-62. PMID: 13937884; PMCID: PMC1932342.

19. Hales CN, Barker DJP. The thrifty phenotype hypothesis. Br Med Bull. 2001;60(1):5–20.
20. Stein Z, Susser M. The Dutch famine, 1944-1945, and the reproductive process. I. Effects on six indices at birth. Pediatr Res. 1975 Feb;9(2):70-6. doi: 10.1203/00006450-197502000-00003. PMID: 1118193.
21. Charney E, Goodman HC, McBride M, Lyon B, Pratt R, Breese B, et al. Childhood antecedents of adult obesity. N Engl J Med. 1976;295(1):6–9.
22. Hofman PL, Cutfield WS, Robinson EM, Bergman RN, Menon RK, Sperling MA, et al. Insulin resistance in short children with intrauterine growth retardation. J Clin Endocrinol Metab. 1997;82(2):402–6.
23. Cianfarani S, Germani D, Branca F. Low birthweight and adult insulin resistance: the "catch-up growth" hypothesis. Arch Dis Child - Fetal Neonatal Ed. 1999;81(1):F71–3.
24. Stöger R. The thrifty epigenotype: an acquired and heritable predisposition for obesity and diabetes? BioEssays. 2008;30(2):156–66.
25. Moisiadis VG, Matthews SG. Glucocorticoids and fetal programming part 1: outcomes. Nat Rev Endocrinol. 2014;10(7):391–402.
26. Moisiadis VG, Matthews SG. Glucocorticoids and fetal programming part 2: mechanisms. Nat Rev Endocrinol. 2014;10(7):403–11.
27. Defronzo RA. Banting Lecture. From the triumvirate to the ominous octet: a new paradigm for the treatment of type 2 diabetes mellitus. Diabetes. 2009;58(4):773–95. https://doi.org/10.2337/db09-9028. PMID: 19336687; PMCID: PMC2661582.
28. Kalra S, Chawla R, Madhu SV. The dirty dozen of diabetes. Indian J Endocrinol Metab. 2013;17(3):367-9. https://doi.org/10.2337/10.4103/2230-8210.111593. PMID: 23869290; PMCID: PMC3712364.
29. Somasundaram NP, Wijesinghe AM. Therapy for type 2 diabetes mellitus: targeting the 'Unlucky Thirteen'. Jacobs J Diabetes Endocrinol. 2016;2(1):12.

# Diagnostic Approaches to Endocrine Disorders

# 8

Kiran Prakash

**Abstract**

Dysfunctional production, secretion or action of hormones results in endocrine disorders. They are diagnosed through a patient's medical history, clinical examinations, and blood tests and further confirmed through dynamic tests, imaging, genetics, and biomarkers. Basal hormone tests that use high-sensitivity immunoassays.

Dynamic tests look at stimulation to find deficiencies and suppression to find excess. Ultrasound, magnetic resonance imaging, and adrenal computed tomography scan help us to identify the structural problems. Genetic tests and biomarkers like copeptin help with subtyping. Multidisciplinary teams use evidence-based guidelines that help in better management of patients.

**Keywords**

Endocrine disorders · Diagnostic evaluation · Dynamic endocrine testing · Genetic testing · Biomarkers · Immunoassays · Magnetic resonance imaging · Adrenal computed tomography

K. Prakash (✉)
Department of Physiology, Government Medical College and Hospital, Sector 32, Chandigarh, India





H. Prabhakar, M. Kaur (eds.), *Brain and Endocrine Crosstalk*, Physiology in Clinical Neurosciences – Brain and Spinal Cord Crosstalks,
https://doi.org/10.1007/978-981-92-0763-3_8

## 8.1 Introduction

Endocrine disorders arise from disruptions in hormone production, secretion, or action. Diagnosis of endocrine disorders primarily requires clinical history, systemic clinical examinations, and basic blood investigations. These further can be substantiated by special stress tests, scans, genetic digs, and sometimes cutting-edge biomarkers [1].

## 8.2 Foundational Diagnostic Framework

A detailed history captures symptoms, for example, fatigue, heat intolerance, polyuria, etc. It also helps us to identify triggers, such as autoimmunity, medications, and neoplasms. The clinical history gets complemented by targeted physical examinations, for example, identification of cushingoid features. Further, biochemical screening employing high-sensitivity immunoassays for basal hormones substantiates our preliminary diagnosis [1, 2].

Various dynamic tests help to evaluate feedback loops. Stimulation tests, for example, cosyntropin for adrenals [3] and GnRH for gonadotropins unmask deficiencies [4], and suppression tests, for example, oral glucose for GH [5] and dexamethasone for cortisol detects hypersecretion [6], aid in diagnosis. Imaging techniques help to detect structural abnormalities and localize pathology, for example, neck ultrasound, pituitary MRI (3T with dynamic sequences), and adrenal CT (non-contrast for adenomas) [7]. Genetic panels (NGS for monogenic disorders) and emerging biomarkers (copeptin for DI and NETest for NENs) refine subtyping [8].

Endocrinologists, imagers, and gene experts work together and stick to guides that are based on solid evidence. They look for smart, affordable ways to get results. AI tools, such as smart algorithms, can find pituitary bumps with almost perfect accuracy.

## 8.3 Thyroid Gland Disorders

The first step in a thyroid status evaluation is assessment of serum thyroid-stimulating hormone (TSH), T3 and T4 levels. A TSH blood test is done first. If the levels are abnormal, a free T4 or T3 test is done. Subclinical hypothyroidism (TSH 4.5–10 mIU/L, normal FT4) warrants screening of thyroid peroxidase antibodies (anti-TPO >35 IU/mL predicts progression). Suppressed TSH and elevated T3 and T4 suggest hyperthyroidism. Uptake scans differentiate toxic nodules (hot) from thyroiditis (low). Resistance syndromes further evaluations. Resistance to Thyroid Hormone Beta presents high FT4/FT3, non-suppressed TSH. Functional assays (T3-responsive reporter genes) corroborate in such cases [9]. Table 8.1 summarizes different thyroid disorders, their biochemical hallmark, and confirmatory tests.

**Table 8.1** Thyroid disorders and their biochemical hallmark and confirmatory tests

| Thyroid disorder | Biochemical hallmark | Confirmatory tests | Genetic/molecular |
|---|---|---|---|
| Primary hypothyroidism | TSH ↑↑, FT4 ↓ | Anti-TPO/TRAb | Polyglandular autoimmunity |
| Graves' hyperthyroidism | TSH ↓↓, FT4/FT3 ↑↑, TRAb ↑ | RAIU high | HLA-DR3 |
| RTHβ | FT4/FT3 ↑, TSH normal/high | THRB NGS | >100 variants |
| MCT8 deficiency | T3 ↑, FT4 ↓, rT3 ↓ | MRI (anterior commissure dysgenesis) | SLC16A2 hemizygous |

*TSH* thyroid-stimulating hormone, *FT4* free thyroxine, *TPO* thyroid peroxidase, *TRAb* thyrotropin receptor antibodies, *FT3* free triiodothyronine, *RAIU* radioactive iodine uptake, *THRB* thyroid hormone receptor beta gene, *NGS* next-generation sequencing, *MRI* magnetic resonance imaging

**Table 8.2** Adrenal disorders, their screening tests, and dynamic confirmation tests

| Adrenal condition | Screening | Dynamic confirmation |
|---|---|---|
| Primary AI | Cortisol <140 nmol/L AM | ACTH stim <500 peak |
| Cushing's syndrome | Late-night salivary cortisol >4 nmol/L ×3 or failed dexamethasone suppression test | Low-dose dexamethasone suppression test/corticotropin-releasing hormone (CRH) stimulation test |
| Primary aldosteronism | Aldosterone-renin ratio >30 | Saline infusion |
| Pheochromocytoma/paraganglioma | Metanephrine levels to twice the upper limit of normal | Clonidine suppression test |

## 8.4 Adrenal Cortex and Medulla Pathology

Adrenal insufficiency (AI) screening: It is done when patients present with unexplained fatigue, weight loss, hypotension, hyponatremia, hypoglycemia, or hyperpigmentation. In initial evaluation early morning serum cortisol is measured. Indeterminate results require confirmatory dynamic testing. Adrenocorticotropic hormone (ACTH) stimulation test is carried out. The measurement of plasma ACTH and electrolytes helps differentiate primary from secondary etiologies. It guides subsequent management of patients [10].

Cushing's syndrome: It requires systemic evaluation for endogenous hypercortisolism and identifying its source. It involves evaluation of late-night salivary cortisol, 24-h urinary free cortisol, or dexamethasone suppression test. At least two abnormal results are required to establish hypercortisolism. Plasma ACTH measurement differentiates ACTH-dependent from ACTH-independent causes. Subsequent tests include high-dose dexamethasone suppression, CRH stimulation, and targeted imaging to localize the source [11].

Table 8.2 summarizes adrenal disorders, their screening tests, and dynamic confirmation tests.

**Table 8.3** Subtypes of diabetes insipidus and its differential diagnosis based on various tests

| DI subtype | WDT urine Osm | Desmopressin response |
|---|---|---|
| Central | <300 milliosmoles per kilogram | >50% ↑ |
| Nephrogenic | <300 milliosmoles per kilogram | <50% ↑ |
| Primary Polydipsia | >300–600 milliosmoles per kilogram | <50% ↑ |

*DI* diabetes insipidus, *WDT* water deprivation test

## 8.5 Pituitary and Hypothalamic Axes

Hypopituitarism secondary to postpartum bleed/trauma: An assessment of basal and dynamic pituitary axes including morning cortisol with ACTH stimulation, free thyroxine with TSH, gonadotropins, and prolactin will be carried out. Further evaluation of water balance tests for diabetes insipidus; deficiencies across anterior hormones are done to confirm hypopituitarism. Magnetic resonance imaging of the sellar region typically demonstrates pituitary infarction with eventual atrophy or an empty sella. Early identification and sequential hormone replacement—prioritizing glucocorticoids before thyroid hormone—are essential to prevent adrenal crisis and optimize outcomes [12].

Acromegaly: Biochemical confirmation is done by assessment of IGF-1. It reflects integrated growth hormone (GH) secretion and is typically elevated in active disease. In case of equivocal IGF-1, an oral glucose tolerance test is performed. High-resolution pituitary magnetic resonance imaging helps to localize a GH-secreting adenoma.

Posterior pituitary pathology usually presents with polyuria/polydipsia. The commonest presentation is in the form of diabetes insipidus [13].

Table 8.3 summarizes the subtypes of diabetes insipidus and its differential diagnosis based on various tests.

## 8.6 Gonadal Dysfunctions and Disorders/Differences of Sex Development

Gonadal dysfunctions and disorders/differences of sex development (DSD) are a group of conditions arising from abnormalities in gonadal differentiation, steroidogenesis, or hormone action. Diagnostic evaluation requires an integrated approach. A detailed phenotypic assessment with endocrine profiling is done. Endocrine profiling includes assessment of gonadotropins, sex steroids, AMH, and inhibin B. Further, cytogenetic and molecular analyses including karyotyping, targeted gene panels, or exome sequencing are done. High-resolution imaging of internal reproductive structures substantiates the diagnosis. Dynamic hormonal testing clarifies the defects in steroid biosynthesis or receptor function [14, 15]. Multidisciplinary interpretation is essential to distinguish primary gonadal failure from central hypogonadism.

**Table 8.4** Modern diagnostic modalities, their underlying technology and key diagnostic applications

| Modality category | Technology/approach | Key diagnostic application |
|---|---|---|
| Advanced biochemical testing | High-sensitivity immunoassays (digital ELISA) | Detection of low-level hormones (ACTH, PTH, GH) |
| | LC–MS/MS steroid profiling | CAH, adrenal tumors, DSD |
| Dynamic functional testing | Time-resolved hormone curves (e.g., late-night cortisol) | Cushing syndrome, adrenal insufficiency |
| | Metabolite-to-precursor ratios (e.g., 17-OHP/S) | Enzyme deficiencies (CAH) |
| Advanced imaging | Dynamic contrast-enhanced MRI | Pituitary microadenomas |
| | Diffusion-weighted MRI | Endocrine tumor characterization (e.g., PanNETs) |
| | Chemical shift MRI | Adrenal incidentalomas |
| Molecular imaging | $^{68}$Ga-DOTATATE PET/CT | Neuroendocrine tumors |
| | $^{11}$C-metomidate PET | Adrenal cortical lesions |
| Genetic diagnostics | Targeted NGS gene panels | MODY, familial endocrine syndromes |
| | Somatic mutation testing | Thyroid, adrenal, pituitary tumors |
| Epigenetic and transcriptomic tools | DNA methylation analysis | Imprinting disorders |
| AI and digital diagnostics | AI-assisted imaging analysis | Thyroid nodules, pituitary adenomas |

*ELISA* enzyme-linked immunosorbent assay, *ACTH* adrenocorticotropic hormone, *PTH* parathyroid hormone, *GH* growth hormone, *LC-MS* liquid chromatography–mass spectrometry, *CAH* congenital adrenal hyperplasia, *DSD* disorders of sex development, *17-OHP/S* 17-hydroxyprogesterone, serum, *MRI* magnetic resonance imaging, *PanNETs* pancreatic neuroendocrine tumors, *PET* positron emission tomography, *CT* computed tomography, *NGS* next-generation sequencing, *MODY* maturity-onset diabetes of the young, *DNA* deoxyribonucleic acid, *AI* artificial intelligence

## 8.7 Technological Advancements

Major technological advancements have aided the precise diagnosis and better management of endocrine disorders. Table 8.4 summarizes the modern diagnostic modalities, their underlying technology, and key diagnostic applications [16–25].

## References


1. Crafa A, Condorelli RA, Cannarella R, Aversa A, Calogero AE, La Vignera S. Physical examination for endocrine diseases: does it still play a role? J Clin Med. 2022;11(9):2598.
2. Spencer-Bonilla G, Singh Ospina N, Rodriguez-Gutierrez R, Brito JP, Iñiguez-Ariza N, Tamhane S, et al. Systematic reviews of diagnostic tests in endocrinology: an audit of methods, reporting, and performance. Endocrine. 2017;57(1):18–34.
3. Jones BR, Shao J, Sanghvi M, Ayala A, Luo R, Wang J. A hybrid IA-LC-MS/MS method for adrenocorticotropic hormone(1-24) to support interpretation of low-dose cosyntropin-stimulation test. Bioanalysis. 2024;16(14):711–20.

4. Sun QH, Zheng Y, Zhang XL, Mu YM. Role of gonadotropin-releasing hormone stimulation test in diagnosing gonadotropin deficiency in both males and females with delayed puberty. Chin Med J (Engl). 2015;128(18):2439–43.
5. Rosario PW, Calsolari MR. Safety and specificity of the growth hormone suppression test in patients with diabetes. Endocrine. 2015;48(1):329–33.
6. Balomenaki M, Margaritopoulos D, Vassiliadi DA, Tsagarakis S. Diagnostic workup of Cushing's syndrome. J Neuroendocrinol. 2022;34(8):e13111.
7. Torigian DA, Li G, Alavi A. The role of CT, MR imaging, and ultrasonography in endocrinology. PET Clin. 2007;2(3):395–408.
8. Newey PJ. Clinical genetic testing in endocrinology: current concepts and contemporary challenges. Clin Endocrinol (Oxf). 2019;91(5):587–607.
9. Li Q, Tang Y, Yu X, Qin G, Tian L, Cheng L, et al. Thyroid function reference intervals by age, sex, and race: a cross-sectional study. Ann Intern Med. 2025;178(7):921–9.
10. Chanson P, Guignat L, Goichot B, Chabre O, Boustani DS, Reynaud R, et al. Group 2: adrenal insufficiency: screening methods and confirmation of diagnosis. Ann Endocrinol (Paris). 2017;78(6):495–511.
11. Findling JW, Raff H. Diagnosis of endocrine disease: differentiation of pathologic/neoplastic hypercortisolism (Cushing's syndrome) from physiologic/non-neoplastic hypercortisolism (formerly known as pseudo-Cushing's syndrome). Eur J Endocrinol. 2017;176(5):R205–16.
12. Higham CE, Johannsson G, Shalet SM. Hypopituitarism. Lancet. 2016;388(10058):2403–15.
13. Tritos NA, Miller KK. Diagnosis and management of pituitary adenomas: a review. JAMA. 2023;329(16):1386–98.
14. Bertelloni S, Tyutyusheva N, Valiani M, D'Alberton F, Baldinotti F, Caligo MA, et al. Disorders/differences of sex development presenting in the newborn with 46, XY karyotype. Front Pediatr. 2021;9:627281.
15. Gomes NL, Batista RL, Nishi MY, Lerário AM, Silva TE, de Moraes Narcizo A, et al. Contribution of clinical and genetic approaches for diagnosing 209 index cases with 46,XY differences of sex development. J Clin Endocrinol Metab. 2022;107(5):e1797–806.
16. Hicks RA, Yee JK, Mao CS, Graham S, Kharrazi M, Lorey F, et al. Precursor-to-product ratios reflect biochemical phenotype in congenital adrenal hyperplasia. Metabolomics. 2014;10(1):123–31.
17. Guo C, Zhuge X, Chen X, Wang Z, Xiao W, Wang Q. Value of diffusion-weighted magnetic resonance imaging in predicting World Health Organization grade in G1/G2 pancreatic neuroendocrine tumors. Oncol Lett. 2017;13(6):4141–6.
18. Li C, Fu Y, Yi X, Guan X, Liu L, Chen BT. Application of radiomics in adrenal incidentaloma: a literature review. Discov Oncol. 2022;13:112.
19. Herrmann K, Czernin J, Wolin EM, Gupta P, Barrio M, Gutierrez A, et al. Impact of 68Ga-DOTATATE PET/CT on the management of neuroendocrine tumors: the referring physician's perspective. J Nucl Med. 2015;56(1):70–5.
20. Bergström M, Juhlin C, Bonasera TA, Sundin A, Rastad J, Akerström G, et al. PET imaging of adrenal cortical tumors with the 11beta-hydroxylase tracer 11C-metomidate. J Nucl Med. 2000;41(2):275–82.
21. Tatsi EB, Kanaka-Gantenbein C, Scorilas A, Chrousos GP, Sertedaki A. Next generation sequencing targeted gene panel in Greek MODY patients increases diagnostic accuracy. Pediatr Diabetes. 2020;21(1):28–39.
22. Moses W, Weng J, Kebebew E. Prevalence, clinicopathologic features, and somatic genetic mutation profile in familial versus sporadic nonmedullary thyroid cancer. Thyroid. 2011;21(4):367–71.
23. Docherty LE, Rezwan FI, Poole RL, Jagoe H, Lake H, Lockett GA, et al. Genome-wide DNA methylation analysis of patients with imprinting disorders identifies differentially methylated regions associated with novel candidate imprinted genes. J Med Genet. 2014;51(4):229–38.
24. Peng S, Liu Y, Lv W, Liu L, Zhou Q, Yang H, et al. Deep learning-based artificial intelligence model to assist thyroid nodule diagnosis and management: a multicentre diagnostic study. Lancet Digit Health. 2021;3(4):e250–9.
25. Li Y, Louie JZ, Burgess TE, Bare LA, McPhaul MJ. Large-scale comparison of two immunoassays for adrenocorticotropic hormone in human plasma. Sci Rep. 2025;15:42854.

# Part II

# Neurophysiology of Endocrine Organs

# Introduction to Neuroendocrinology

9

Kiran Prakash

**Abstract**

Neuroendocrinology deals with the integrated functioning of the nervous and endocrine systems in maintaining homeostasis and coordinating adaptive responses. This chapter outlines the fundamental concepts of neuroendocrine regulation, emphasizing the pivotal role of the hypothalamus in linking neural signals with hormonal secretion. Major hypothalamic–pituitary axes, including the adrenal, gonadal, thyroid, and growth hormone axes, are described to illustrate systemic control of stress, metabolism, reproduction, and growth. Interactions at the cellular level involving neurotransmitters, hormones, shared receptors, and intracellular signaling pathways are discussed along with feedback mechanisms that ensure physiological stability. The chapter also highlights integration with the immune and autonomic nervous systems and briefly reviews the clinical implications of neuroendocrine dysregulation.

**Keywords**

Neuroendocrinology · Hypothalamus · Hypothalamic–pituitary axis · Homeostasis · Feedback regulation · Stress response · Autonomic nervous system · Immune–neuroendocrine interaction

## 9.1 Neuroendocrinology: Definition and Its Importance

Neuroendocrinology is the study of brain and hormonal interactions to keep the body balanced. It explores the bidirectional interactions between neurons—primarily in the brain—and endocrine glands, which secrete hormones that influence a multitude of bodily functions from growth and development to metabolism, stress response, reproduction, circadian rhythms, and social behaviors. In recent decades,

K. Prakash (✉)
Department of Physiology, Government Medical College and Hospital, Chandigarh, India



H. Prabhakar, M. Kaur (eds.), *Brain and Endocrine Crosstalk*, Physiology in Clinical Neurosciences – Brain and Spinal Cord Crosstalks,
https://doi.org/10.1007/978-981-92-0763-3_9

the field has advanced quickly, driven by major progress in molecular biology, genetics, electrophysiology, and imaging. These tools have allowed researchers to uncover the intricate mechanisms that shape neuroendocrine signaling [1, 2].

Neuroendocrinology was formally established with the discovery that the brain controls the pituitary gland through the release of specialized neurohormones. This principle, demonstrated through pioneering work on the hypothalamic–pituitary axis, laid the foundation for the field. The axis shows how the hypothalamus produces hormones that regulate the pituitary, which in turn directs activity in organs and tissues throughout the body. Through these pathways, the nervous system can influence distant systems such as the adrenal, thyroid, reproductive, and metabolic axes. In return, hormones from these organs feed back to the brain, shaping neural activity, behavior, and cognition [2, 3].

The importance of neuroendocrinology has become especially pronounced with the recognition that virtually all major physiological and psychological processes—such as stress adaptation, appetite regulation, reproductive cycles, and social affiliation—depend on neuroendocrine signaling networks. For instance, the neuroendocrine stress axis—better known as the hypothalamic–pituitary–adrenal (HPA) axis—helps the body adapt to challenges. It translates the brain's perception of stress into hormonal signals that influence immunity, metabolism, and behavior [4]. Additionally, neuropeptides like oxytocin and vasopressin serve dual roles as neurotransmitters and hormones, mediating social behaviors, emotional bonding, and pain perception [5].

Contemporary neuroendocrinology is highly interdisciplinary and draws upon advances in neuroscience, molecular biology, computational analysis, genetics, and behavioral sciences to elucidate the dynamic interplay between hormones and brain function. Today, research extends beyond the classic systems like the hypothalamic–pituitary–gonadal and HPA axes to examine how neuroendocrine signals interact with circadian rhythms, feeding, and brain development. Large-scale efforts, such as the BRAIN Initiative, highlight the growing urgency to understand how hormones shape the neural circuits that drive cognition, emotion, and vulnerability to disease [6].

For scientists, neuroendocrinology is an exciting and rapidly growing field, where understanding how the brain and hormones interact is paving the way for new treatments for neurological, psychiatric, and endocrine disorders. Its integrative nature exemplifies the complexity of biological regulation—illuminating how the central nervous system and endocrine glands cooperate to enable organisms to adapt, survive, and thrive in a changing environment.

## 9.2 Interactions Between the Nervous and Endocrine System

The nervous and endocrine systems work together to maintain the homeostasis. Their interactions range from large-scale feedback loops across multiple organs to finely tuned cellular and molecular processes that help the body adapt to both internal changes and external challenges.

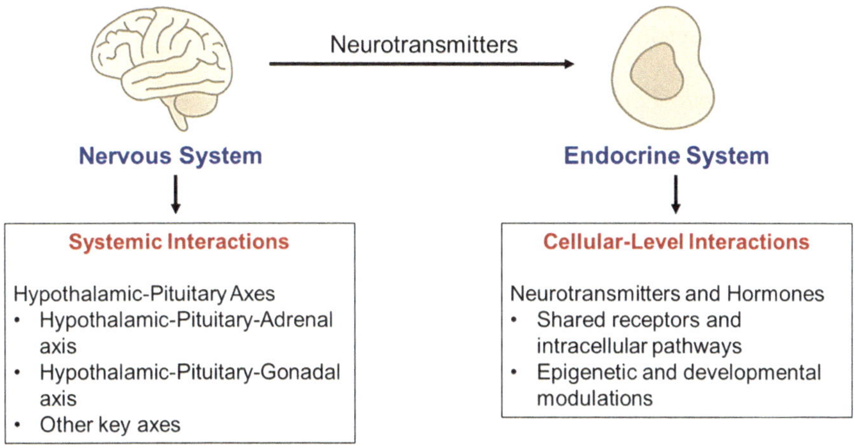


**Fig. 9.1** Interactions between nervous and endocrine systems

The neuroendocrine system encompasses the complex bidirectional communication between the central nervous system (CNS), peripheral nervous system, and various endocrine glands. This communication is essential for coordinating signals that control growth, metabolism, stress, reproduction, energy use, immune function, and even how behavior adapts to changes in the environment [7–9].

Neurons and endocrine glands utilize molecular messengers—neurotransmitters and hormones—to mediate systemic and tissue-specific effects. The hypothalamus serves as a central regulatory node, linking neural circuits with hormonal control through releasing factors that act on the pituitary gland and, subsequently, the peripheral endocrine organs. Feedback from these organs communicates the physiological state back to the CNS, closing the regulatory loop [10].

The interactions of nervous and endocrine system occur both at system and at cellular levels (Fig. 9.1).

## 9.3 Systemic Interactions

### 9.3.1 Hypothalamic–Pituitary Axes

- *Hypothalamic–Pituitary–Adrenal (HPA) Axis*

The HPA axis is the body's core stress-response system. When stress is detected, neurons in the hypothalamus release signaling molecules—CRF and vasopressin—into the pituitary. This triggers the pituitary to release ACTH, which then stimulates the adrenal glands to produce glucocorticoids, mainly cortisol in humans. Glucocorticoids mobilize energy, modulate immune responses, and provide negative feedback to both the hypothalamus and pituitary, modulating the response and preventing over-activation. Disruption of this loop is implicated in mood disorders and metabolic syndromes [11].

- *Hypothalamic–Pituitary–Gonadal (HPG) Axis*

In reproductive regulation, GnRH released by the hypothalamus stimulates the pituitary to secrete luteinizing hormone (LH) and follicle-stimulating hormone (FSH), which then act on the gonads to drive sex hormone production and gametogenesis. Sex steroids (estrogen and testosterone) provide feedback to both brain and pituitary, affecting not only reproduction but also immunity, brain development, and behavior [11].

- *Other key axes*

*Hypothalamic–Pituitary–Thyroid (HPT) Axis* regulates metabolism and growth through thyroid hormone synthesis [12].

*Hypothalamic–Growth Hormone Axis* coordinates somatic growth and metabolic processes [13].

Together, these systems allow the brain and hormones to work in sync, using feedback loops to help the body adapt to both internal needs and external challenges.

## 9.4 Cellular-Level Interactions

Neurotransmitters are chemical messengers released from nerve endings that act on nearby neurons or cells, while hormones travel through the bloodstream to affect organs and tissues farther away. Many peptide hormones (e.g., oxytocin and vasopressin) serve both as CNS neurotransmitters and as systemic hormones, producing coordinated effects on behavior and physiology [14].

***Shared Receptors and Intracellular Pathways*** Neurons, glial cells, and endocrine cells all carry receptors for each other's signals. This allows messengers such as glucocorticoids, estrogens, catecholamines, and neuropeptides to influence gene activity, shape synaptic connections, and regulate secretion at the cellular level [15, 16].

Feedback regulation occurs at both the gene transcription and protein activity levels, impacting everything from synapse formation to metabolic enzyme function.

***Epigenetic and Developmental Modulation*** Early life experiences, such as maternal care, alter the expression of glucocorticoid receptors in key brain regions through epigenetic changes (methylation/acetylation), influencing stress resilience throughout life [17].

Epigenetic modifications of stress-response genes (e.g., CRF and BDNF) play central roles in mood disorders and adaptation [18].

## 9.5 Bidirectional Feedback: Integration of Systems

### 9.5.1 Immune System and Neuroendocrine Integration

Immune cells like lymphocytes and macrophages have receptors for neurotransmitters and hormones, while the brain and endocrine organs, in turn, carry receptors for immune signals such as cytokines and growth factors [19].

The HPA axis and sympathetic nervous system can suppress or enhance immunity, with stress often leading to immunosuppression, increased susceptibility to infection, and modulation of inflammation. Cytokines released during immune responses reach the brain, influencing neuroendocrine activity and behavior (e.g., sickness behavior and mood disorders) [20].

### 9.5.2 Autonomic Nervous System and Endocrine Output

The autonomic nervous system (ANS) and endocrine output form a highly integrated regulatory network that orchestrates organismal homeostasis under both basal and stress-challenged conditions. Effector pathways of the ANS—the sympathetic and parasympathetic branches—innervate peripheral endocrine organs (e.g., adrenal medulla, pancreatic islets, and ovaries) and key hypothalamic centers such as the paraventricular nucleus of the hypothalamus (PVN), which contains both neuroendocrine and autonomic preganglionic neurons [21]. Through these connections, autonomic outflow directly modulates hormone secretion (catecholamines, insulin, cortisol, and gonadal steroids), and reciprocally, hormonal signals (glucocorticoids, insulin, and gonadotropins) dynamically calibrate autonomic tone via central feedback loops. For example, sympathetic input sensitizes adrenal cortical responses to anterior pituitary ACTH and modifies ovarian sensitivity in PCOS [22]. Moreover, the ANS interprets afferent hormonal and nutrient signals (e.g., via vagal afferents) to adjust systemic metabolism: An emerging review emphasizes afferent–efferent loops by which the ANS regulates energy and glucose homeostasis, while endocrine feedback modifies central autonomic circuits [23]. Thus, the ANS and endocrine systems act as a dual-modality controller: The ANS provides rapid neural modulation, and the endocrine axis provides sustained hormonal modulation. Dysregulation of this interface underlies pathophysiologies such as metabolic syndrome, stress-related disorders, and autonomic–endocrine dysfunctions.

## 9.6 Clinical and Therapeutic Implications

Dysregulation of neuroendocrine interactions underlies a wide range of disorders: psychiatric illness (depression and PTSD), metabolic syndrome, autoimmune and inflammatory diseases, reproductive disorders, and aging-related conditions [24, 25].

Interventions targeting these systems include glucocorticoid administration for PTSD, hormone replacement, neuromodulation, lifestyle modification (stress reduction and nutrition), and emerging molecular therapeutics [26, 27].

Understanding cell- and circuit-level mechanisms is paving the way for precision medicine approaches in neuroendocrinology.

## 9.7 Conclusion

The nervous and endocrine systems are closely linked, working together from the level of whole-body responses down to signals inside individual cells. By coordinating their actions, they allow the body to adapt quickly and flexibly to changes both inside and outside the body. Advances in genomics, systems biology, imaging, and molecular neuroscience are continually refining our understanding of these dynamic networks.

The future of neuroendocrinology lies in unravelling even more precise molecular, genetic, and circuit-level interactions that mediate resilience, vulnerability, and disease development. Continued research will inform novel interventions for neuropsychiatric, endocrine, immune, and metabolic disorders, emphasizing the importance of integrative biological regulation for human health.

## References

1. Vaudry H. Editorial: trends in neuroendocrinology. Front Endocrinol (Lausanne). 2016;7:41.
2. Russell JA. Fifty years of advances in neuroendocrinology. Brain Neurosci Adv. 2018;2:2398212818812014.
3. Kaiser UB. Editorial: Advances in neuroscience: the brain initiative and implications for neuroendocrinology. Mol Endocrinol. 2014;28(10):1589–91.
4. Smith SM, Vale WW. The role of the hypothalamic-pituitary-adrenal axis in neuroendocrine responses to stress. Dialogues Clin Neurosci. 2006;8(4):383–95.
5. Rigney N, de Vries GJ, Petrulis A, Young LJ. Oxytocin, vasopressin, and social behavior: from neural circuits to clinical opportunities. Endocrinology. 2022;163(9):bqac111.
6. Ecker JR, Geschwind DH, Kriegstein AR, Ngai J, Osten P, Polioudakis D, et al. The BRAIN Initiative Cell Census Consortium: lessons learned toward generating a comprehensive BRAIN cell atlas. Neuron. 2017;96(3):542–57.
7. Kalra SP, Kalra PS. Neuroendocrine control of energy homeostasis: update on new insights. Prog Brain Res. 2010;181:17–33.
8. Padmanabhan V, Sharma TP. Neuroendocrine vs. paracrine control of follicle-stimulating hormone. Arch Med Res. 2001;32(6):533–43.
9. Quijije N. Updates in the neuroendocrinology of stress and its clinical management. Curr Opin Endocrinol Diabetes Obes. 2015;22(4):319–24.

10. Acher R, Chauvet J. The neurohypophysial endocrine regulatory cascade: precursors, mediators, receptors, and effectors. Front Neuroendocrinol. 1995;16(3):237–89.
11. Oyola MG, Handa RJ. Hypothalamic-pituitary-adrenal and hypothalamic-pituitary-gonadal axes: sex differences in regulation of stress responsivity. Stress. 2017;20(5):476–94.
12. Mullur R, Liu YY, Brent GA. Thyroid hormone regulation of metabolism. Physiol Rev. 2014;94(2):355–82.
13. Ghigo E, Arvat E, Gianotti L, Lanfranco F, Broglio F, Aimaretti G, et al. Hypothalamic growth hormone-insulin-like growth factor-I axis across the human life span. J Pediatr Endocrinol Metab. 2000;13(Suppl 6):1493–502.
14. Benarroch EE. Oxytocin and vasopressin: social neuropeptides with complex neuromodulatory functions. Neurology. 2013 Apr 16;80(16):1521–8.
15. Jauregui-Huerta F, Ruvalcaba-Delgadillo Y, Gonzalez-Castañeda R, Garcia-Estrada J, Gonzalez-Perez O, Luquin S. Responses of glial cells to stress and glucocorticoids. Curr Immunol Rev. 2010;6(3):195–204.
16. McEwen BS, Akama KT, Spencer-Segal JL, Milner TA, Waters EM. Estrogen effects on the brain: actions beyond the hypothalamus via novel mechanisms. Behav Neurosci. 2012;126(1):4–16.
17. Palma-Gudiel H, Córdova-Palomera A, Eixarch E, Deuschle M, Fañanás L. Maternal psychosocial stress during pregnancy alters the epigenetic signature of the glucocorticoid receptor gene promoter in their offspring: a meta-analysis. Epigenetics. 2015;10(10):893–902.
18. Miao Z, Wang Y, Sun Z. The relationships between stress, mental disorders, and epigenetic regulation of BDNF. Int J Mol Sci. 2020;21(4):1375.
19. Taub DD. Neuroendocrine interactions in the immune system. Cell Immunol. 2008;252(1–2):1–6.
20. Marcolongo-Pereira C, Castro FC de AQ, Barcelos RM, Chiepe KCMB, Rossoni Junior JV, Ambrosio RP, et al. Neurobiological mechanisms of mood disorders: stress vulnerability and resilience. Front Behav Neurosci. 2022;16:1006836.
21. Sladek CD, Michelini LC, Stachenfeld NS, Stern JE, Urban JH. Endocrine-autonomic linkages. Compr Physiol. 2015;5(3):1281–323.
22. Engeland WC. Sensitization of endocrine organs to anterior pituitary hormones by the autonomic nervous system. Handb Clin Neurol. 2013;117:37–44.
23. Hyun U, Sohn JW. Autonomic control of energy balance and glucose homeostasis. Exp Mol Med. 2022;54(4):370–6.
24. Yehuda R. Advances in understanding neuroendocrine alterations in PTSD and their therapeutic implications. Ann N Y Acad Sci. 2006;1071:137–66.
25. Cozma D, Siatra P, Bornstein SR, Steenblock C. Sensitivity of the neuroendocrine stress axis in metabolic diseases. Horm Metab Res. 2024;56(1):65–77.
26. Bidlingmaier M, Gleeson H, Latronico AC, Savage MO. Applying precision medicine to the diagnosis and management of endocrine disorders. Endocr Connect. 2022;11(10):e220177.
27. Florido A, Velasco ER, Monari S, Cano M, Cardoner N, Sandi C, et al. Glucocorticoid-based pharmacotherapies preventing PTSD. Neuropharmacology. 2023;224:109344.

# Neural Regulation of Endocrine System 10

Mahesh Arjundan Gadhvi and Shival Srivastav

**Abstract**

'Neuroendocrinology' describes the branch of physiology that describes the handshake between the nervous and endocrine systems. It has been observed that these two systems are intricately connected and play important roles in maintenance of homeostasis. Both 'top down' and 'bottom-up' signalling pathways have been worked out that underscore the interaction between the neural and endocrine systems. In the present review, we will discuss this neuroendocrine control of body functions with emphasis of the role of hypothalamus and autonomic nervous system.

**Keywords**

Neuroendocrinology · Hypothalamus · Functions of hypothalamus · Autonomic nervous system

## 10.1 Part I: Background

### 10.1.1 The Foundations of Neuroendocrinology: The Work of Geoffrey Harris

The seminal work of Geoffrey Harris laid the foundations of neuroendocrinology, by describing the intricate connections between the hypothalamus and the pituitary gland. He, along with John Green [1, 2], described the anatomical details of the portal system connecting the pituitary and hypothalamus. This was followed by a detailed experimental work on the role of hypothalamic-pituitary axis on the control

M. A. Gadhvi · S. Srivastav (✉)
AIIMS Jodhpur, Jodhpur, India
e-mail: gadhvima@aiimsjodhpur.edu.in; srivastavs@aiimsjodhpur.edu.in


H. Prabhakar, M. Kaur (eds.), *Brain and Endocrine Crosstalk*, Physiology in Clinical Neurosciences – Brain and Spinal Cord Crosstalks,
https://doi.org/10.1007/978-981-92-0763-3_10

of different bodily functions in diverse animal models—ranging from rat to Macau monkey [3–5].

Harris and colleagues described the requirements for a chemical substance to act as a releasing hormone based on three cardinal qualities—presence in local hypophysial circulation in elaborate amounts, change in concentration of this factor after stimulation of hypothalamic neurons, and ability of the substance to affect the functions of the adenohypophysis [6]. Harris described the term 'releasing factors' for such substances, and the terminology has been widely accepted decades after his work.

Building on this foundation, Harris also described three properties that were fundamental to our understanding of how hypothalamus controls the pituitary gland. These were as follows:

(a) Presence of releasing hormones that provide chemical link between hypothalamus and pituitary
(b) Discrete localization of function in different hypothalamic areas
(c) Pituitary stalk acts as the 'final common pathway' for pituitary gland.

The contributions of Geoffrey Harris are well described in excellent reviews by Watts [6], Raisman [7], and Silver and colleagues [8].

### 10.1.2 Three Key Components of Neuroendocrinology

Hypothalamus plays a key role in neuroendocrine functions of the body. It serves as an integrator of diverse physiological signals—ranging from stress to thirst and hunger and circadian fluctuations. It is anatomically as well as physiologically connected to the pituitary—a pea-sized gland housed in Sella turcica. The pituitary secretes many hormones through its two segments—anterior and posterior pituitary. While the anterior pituitary primarily releases 'stimulating hormones' that stimulate endocrine glands to secrete their individual hormones into the blood stream, the posterior pituitary releases 'anti-diuretic' hormone (vasopressin) and oxytocin—which are fundamental to maintenance of body osmolality via regulation of urinary volume and lactation, respectively.

The hypothalamus also controls the autonomic nervous system (ANS), which serves to regulate endocrine responses via multiple effector systems.

## 10.2 Part II: Hypothalamus—The Seat of Neuroendocrine Functions

### 10.2.1 Background

The hypothalamus, a small structure located at the base of the brain, has numerous crucial multisystem functions to perform, including the regulation of endocrine hormones and the control of circadian rhythms, as well as the regulation of thirst, hunger, and many other bodily functions. Through its neuroendocrine structure, the hypothalamus bridges the neural and endocrine systems. Most of its effects on endocrine organs are mediated through the effect on the pituitary gland, which in turn regulates other endocrine glands [9].

Before delving into the endocrine functions of the hypothalamus, let us first understand its anatomy and various functions.

### 10.2.2 Anatomy of the Hypothalamus

The hypothalamus is developed in the embryo from the most anterior portion of the neural tube. The diencephalon makes most of the part of the hypothalamus, except the preoptic area, which is derived from the telencephalon [10].

The hypothalamus is located near the thalamus and the floor of the fourth ventricle. The optic chiasma forms its anterior boundary, while posteriorly it is bound by the mammillary body and laterally by the optic nerve. Around 12 different nuclei are present in the hypothalamus, which can be divided into anterior, posterior, and tuberal regions. Key hypothalamic nuclei include the suprachiasmatic nucleus, the preoptic nucleus, and the paraventricular nucleus [11].

It is clear from Table 10.1 that the hypothalamus is involved in numerous control mechanisms that maintain homeostasis. We will explore the most important function of the hypothalamus, which is regulating endocrine hormones, primarily through the pituitary gland.

**Table 10.1** Hypothalamic nuclei and their main functions

| Hypothalamic nucleus | Function |
|---|---|
| Preoptic nucleus | Controls autonomic functions and sexual behaviour |
| Suprachiasmatic nucleus | Circadian rhythm |
| Anterior nucleus | Thermoregulation |
| Paraventricular nucleus | Growth regulation |
| Dorsomedial nucleus | Feeding centres |
| Ventromedial | Controls appetite and satiety |
| Arcuate nucleus | Growth hormone synthesis, appetite regulation |
| Supraoptic nucleus | Synthesis of vasopressin |
| Mammillary bodies | Memory formation |
| Tuberomammillary nucleus | Role in memory and arousal |
| Posterior hypothalamic nucleus | Body temperature regulation |

### 10.2.3 Endocrine Functions of the Hypothalamus

#### 10.2.3.1 GHRH (Growth Hormone-Releasing Hormone)

GHRH is released from the arcuate nucleus of the hypothalamus. As its name denotes, it stimulates the anterior pituitary to release growth hormone. GHRH is stored in the medial eminence and released through the portal system into the anterior pituitary and stimulates somatotrophs to release growth hormone. GHRH exerts this effect by G protein-coupled receptors over somatotrophs, and point mutation in GHRH receptors causes pituitary hypoplasia in experimental settings [12].

In addition to its effect on anterior pituitary, GHRH has widespread actions in the body where it causes cell proliferation and differentiation. GHRH causes pancreatic beta cell growth and promotes wound healing, anti-inflammatory actions, and endometrial cell proliferation [13].

#### 10.2.3.2 GnRH (Gonadotropin-Releasing Hormone)

Gonadotropins, follicle-stimulating hormone (FSH), and Luteinizing hormone (LH) are vital for reproductive physiology. Both FSH and LH are synthesized and released by the anterior pituitary, but their release is regulated by the hypothalamus through GnRH. Unlike other hypothalamic hormone-secreting cells, GnRH cells are scattered throughout the gland [14].

One peculiar feature of GnRH is its pulsatile release. GnRH release does not start in the early years of life, but rather at around 13–16 years of age, when GnRH release begins in pulses, lasting 1–2 min and followed by a period of no release for 1 h. This pulsatile release is the reason for the stimulation of gonadotropin release [14].

Extensive research began in 2003 to determine the reason behind the hypothalamus's intrinsic ability to secrete GnRH in a pulsatile manner. Loss-of-function mutation of GPR54 (G protein-coupled receptor) is responsible for hypogonadotropic hypogonadism, and the ligand for GPR54 is known as kisspeptin or metastin. Neurons that secrete kisspeptin are present in the arcuate nucleus, which lies near the median eminence. Attachment of kisspeptin to the GPR54 is responsible for the pulsatile release of GnRH [15].

Another substance related to the GnRH pulse generator was discovered by Topaloglu et al. in 2009, known as neurokinin B. A loss-of-function mutation of neurokinin B also produces the same symptoms as those of kisspeptin. The neurons for neurokinin B are also present in the arcuate nucleus, alongside kisspeptin neurons, and regulate GnRH secretion [16].

Goodman et al. in 2007 expressed another opioid that is co-expressed with neurokinin B and kisspeptin in the arcuate nucleus, which is known as dynorphin [17]. It is also responsible for the GnRH pulse generator. All three peptides are together known as KNDs. Dynorphin is inhibitory, while neurokinin B is stimulatory for the release of GnRH, whereas the ultimate GnRH release is because of kisspeptin released from the arcuate nucleus.

#### 10.2.3.3 Oxytocin

Oxytocin is one of the hormones synthesized directly by the hypothalamus and transported to the posterior pituitary gland, where it is stored in vesicles and released into the bloodstream when stimulation arrives. Oxytocin is important in the milk ejection reflex and plays a central role in uterine contractions during labour.

With these effects on reproductive organs, oxytocin is also very important for social cognition. Studies found lower levels of oxytocin in suicide survivors and happy social individuals with higher levels of oxytocin. It also influences social attachment and parenting behaviours [18]. Patients with hypothalamic injury have lower levels of oxytocin and have symptoms of cognitive decline, but these symptoms are reversible with oxytocin therapy [19].

The neurons for the synthesis are located in the supraoptic and paraventricular nuclei of the hypothalamus. They are magnocellular neurons and are located near the neurons for vasopressin release [18]. Magnocellular neurons project into the posterior pituitary. In contrast, parvocellular neurons, which also release vasopressin, secrete oxytocin and vasopressin to other areas of the brain, such as the anterior pituitary, amygdala, and brainstem [20].

#### 10.2.3.4 Vasopressin

Vasopressin, also known as antidiuretic hormone, is synthesized by the hypothalamus, along with oxytocin. Vasopressin acts on the kidney and regulates water reabsorption from the collecting duct, which helps to maintain water balance in the body. Vasopressin also acts on blood vessels, constricting the arteries to regulate blood pressure. Damage to the hypothalamus can cause diabetes insipidus, a condition in which the decreased synthesis of vasopressin results in increased water loss from the kidneys [21].

Like oxytocin, vasopressin is also synthesized in magnocellular neurons of the supraoptic and paraventricular nuclei of the hypothalamus and stored in axon terminals present in the posterior pituitary [22].

#### 10.2.3.5 Thyrotropin-Releasing Hormone (TRH)

One of the most vital hormones for maintaining homeostasis is the thyroid hormone, which is synthesized by the thyroid gland. TRH is a tripeptide also called thyroliberin. For the regulation of thyroid hormone in the blood, thyroid-stimulating hormone is released from the anterior pituitary, which in turn is regulated by thyrotropin-releasing hormone, synthesized by the hypothalamus. These studies demonstrate the role of TRH in regulating thyroid hormone levels.

TRH acts by TRH receptors, which are G protein-coupled receptors [23]. TRH receptors are also present on the cells that synthesize prolactin. Studies found an increased level of prolactin in patients with higher TRH levels [24].

In addition to its effect on thyroid hormone synthesis, TRH is also involved in water regulation, feeding, and thermogenesis [25]. It has a role in the recurrence of depression in the long run [26]. Non-thyroid function of TRH does not stop here. Studies have shown the effect of TRH on the functions of the cerebellum.

Administration of TRH is associated with improvement in ataxic gait. Its effect in the cerebellum is through cyclic GMP [27].

#### 10.2.3.6 Corticotropin-Releasing Hormone

Corticotropin-releasing hormone (CRH) is released from the hypothalamus and is an important component of the hypothalamic-pituitary-adrenal axis. Synthesized from paraventricular cells of the hypothalamus, it reaches the anterior pituitary through portal circulation and causes the release of adrenocorticotropic hormone, which in turn stimulates the adrenal gland and thus regulates the release of hormones related to stress from the adrenal gland [28].

Other than the hypothalamus, the placenta is the site from which CRH is released during pregnancy. Its release starts in the first trimester and gradually increases until the third trimester, when its levels are the highest. Its level in blood remains high and does not show diurnal change or change during stress [29]. During pregnancy, it is believed to have an important role in foetal maturation and the timing of delivery [30].

In addition to its effect on the HPA axis, CRH also exhibits some indirect anti-inflammatory properties. CRH activates the HPA axis, which in turn elevates cortisol levels, a hormone with anti-inflammatory activity. Interleukin-6 is believed to activate the HPA axis. CRH receptors are present on lymphocytes, and the presence of immunogenic CRH in the synovial fluid of rheumatoid arthritis patients suggests its role in immunity [31].

#### 10.2.3.7 Dopamine

The hypothalamus synthesizes and releases dopamine, a neurotransmitter, to inhibit prolactin release from the anterior pituitary and thus plays an important part in prolactin regulation. The dorsomedian hypothalamic arcuate nucleus contains tuberoinfundibular dopamine neurons, which are responsible for the synthesis of neuroendocrine dopamine. From portal circulation, dopamine acts on the anterior pituitary [32].

### 10.2.4 Non-hormonal Functions of the Hypothalamus

The hypothalamus has a profound effect on the pituitary gland, regulating most of the pituitary hormone synthesis and release. But there are many important and vital functions of the body other than hormones, which the hypothalamus regulates.

#### 10.2.4.1 Temperature Regulation

The body's internal temperature remains in a very narrow range, and cellular chemical reactions function efficiently in this narrow range of temperature. The anterior nucleus is responsible for regulating body temperature [33]. Temperature is sensed by thermoreceptors, and the information is conveyed to the anterior hypothalamus, which sends signals to regulate temperature [34].

#### 10.2.4.2 Appetite and Hunger

Fasting or feeding the state has a direct impact on our day-to-day functioning and the perception of hunger and satiety, which is regulated by the hypothalamus. Ghrelin, released from the gut, and leptin, released from adipose tissue, act on the hypothalamus. Ghrelin acts on growth hormone secretagogue receptors in the lateral hypothalamus and paraventricular nucleus to increase food intake [35].

#### 10.2.4.3 Circadian Rhythm

Circadian changes and the environment reflect in our body, and the body adjusts its functions during day and night. The suprachiasmatic nucleus of the hypothalamus is a key component of the circadian rhythm [36].

#### 10.2.4.4 Sleep and Wakefulness

The tuberomammillary nucleus, the lateral hypothalamus, and the orexin-secreting neurons all play a role in regulating wakefulness. In addition to this, the areas of the brainstem responsible for wakefulness send their signals to the cortex, which then passes through the hypothalamus. Preoptic neurons contain some sleep-promoting neurons, which are in turn regulated by neurotransmitters released during the arousal state. Hence, mutual activation and inactivation between these two systems help induce sleep and wakefulness [37].

## 10.3 Part III: ANS as a Neuroendocrine Regulator

Autonomic nervous system (ANS), previously considered a non-descript part of the nervous system, has emerged as an important player in bodily functions. Its innervation spans almost all important organ systems, and pathological changes in ANS have been implicated in multiple disorders spanning almost all organ systems [38–41].

### 10.3.1 History of the ANS

The earliest description of the ANS has been observed in writings by Galen, where peripheral ganglia have been described in gross dissections. Major strides were made in nineteenth century, wherein works of Gaskell, Langley, Bernard, and Cannon laid the foundations of the present understanding of ANS. JN Langley is credited with coining of the term ANS in the late 1890s. Autonomic neurotransmission was described in the seminal works of Elliott, Dale, and Loewi. Sir Henry Hariett Dale is credited with coining the terms nicotinic and muscarinic, whereas Otto Loewi described the release of '*vagusstoff*' from vagal nerve endings in his amphibian experimental setups. A detailed history of the ANS is described elsewhere [42–44].

## 10.3.2 Overview of the ANS

The ANS consists of two mutually antagonistic limbs—the sympathetic nervous system (SNS) and the parasympathetic nervous system (PNS). Enteric nervous system, present in the wall of the gastrointestinal tract, is also considered as a limb of the ANS. ANS controls all major body systems and helps regulate bodily functions.

Sympathetic nervous system (SNS) is also termed as the 'thoraco-lumbar' outflow, since the preganglionic segments of this limb are located in the thoracic and lumbar segments of the spinal cord. The pre-ganglionic fibres are relatively smaller in length, and they synapse close to the spinal cord in the pre- and para-vertebral ganglia. These ganglia constitute the sympathetic chain and give rise to the post ganglionic fibres that innervate multiple organs.

The parasympathetic division is known as the 'cranio-sacral' division, since it originates from the cranial nerves (III, VII, IX, and X) and sacral segments of spinal cord (S2–S4). Here the preganglionic fibres are longer than those seen in SNS, and they synapse in the ganglia that are located close to the effector organs. Hence, the postganglionic fibres are smaller in length, due to close proximity between the organs and the ganglia.

There are two key neurotransmitter systems in the ANS. Acetylcholine (ACh) is present in the preganglionic fibres of both PNS and SNS and all postganglionic endings of the PNS. Sympathetic cholinergic fibres are also observed in the sweat glands, ACh being the notable exception here.

ACh acts via two key receptor systems—nicotinic and muscarinic receptors. Nicotinic receptors are ligand-gated ion channels, wherein binding of ACh leads to ion influx and generation of potential. Muscarinic receptors are primarily G protein-coupled receptors (GPCRs) that act via second messenger pathways.

SNS has norepinephrine (NE) as the main neurotransmitter. In addition, epinephrine is also poured directly into the bloodstream by adrenal medulla. Two key receptor systems in the SNS are α and β. These receptors are GPCRs, which act via the second messenger signalling. Autonomic neurons also exhibit non-adrenergic and non-cholinergic transmission, wherein neuropeptide Y, adenosine triphosphate, and other diverse neurotransmitters may be involved in signalling.

## 10.3.3 The Interaction Between ANS and Pancreas

The pancreas—through its exocrine and endocrine parts—plays an important role in regulating the handling of different nutrients that are key to body functions. While the exocrine segment releases key enzymes that digest carbohydrates, lipids, and proteins, the endocrine segment of the gland releases insulin and glucagon that help regulate the levels of glucose in the blood stream. Glucose is utilized by the body as a key energy substrate and is fundamental to different body functions. The body devotes considerable resources to maintain blood glucose levels and has elaborate mechanisms to prevent hypo- and hyper-glycaemia. This homeostasis is brought about by a delicate interplay between levels of insulin and glucagon—two key hormones secreted by endocrine pancreas. Therefore, while the exocrine part of the pancreas ensures availability of nutrients through the gastro-intestinal tract, the endocrine part of the gland facilitates optimum levels of glucose in the bloodstream for survival.

The established understanding has been that islets of Langerhans present in the pancreas have the ability to respond to fluctuating glucose levels in our blood stream in an autonomous manner. However, increasing evidence points out that this activity is not entirely autonomous at the level of the gland and the brain helps fine tune the levels of glucose in the body.

Autonomic innervation of the pancreas was described as early as 1860s by Langerhans himself, which was substantiated in multiple studies later on [45]. We now know that pancreas is densely innervated by both the sympathetic and parasympathetic nervous system. These nerves enter the core of the islets and form multiple intra pancreatic ganglia in the immediate vicinity of the cell clusters [46]. In addition, neuronal projections from the enteric nervous system have also been identified. Sympathetic fibres arise from Intermediolateral column of the spinal cord, via the celiac and superior mesenteric ganglia. Parasympathetic fibres originate from dorsal motor nucleus of the X cranial nerve, vagus. In addition to cholinergic innervation, PNS also communicates via vasoactive intestinal polypeptide (VIP) and gastrin releasing peptide (GRP). The hierarchy of ANS supply to the pancreas is summarized in Fig. 10.1.

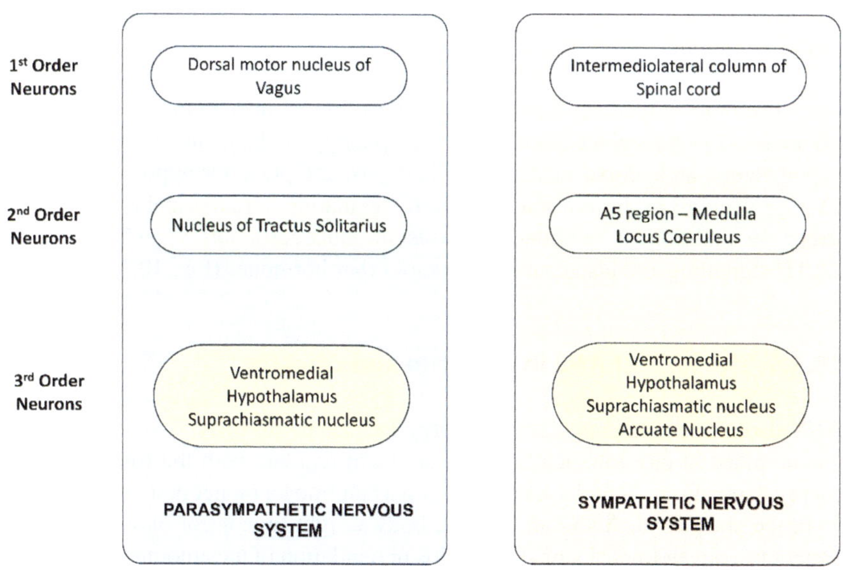


**Fig. 10.1** Hierarchy of autonomic neural supply to the pancreas. The first-, second-, and third-order neurons of sympathetic and parasympathetic nervous system are shown. (Figure is based on information provided in Ref. [47])

By virtue of hierarchical connections between the nervous system and pancreas, a coordinated response is shown to perturbations in blood glucose levels. Glucose sensing abilities are observed in key neurons located at first, second, and third order of the hierarchy. The absence of blood-brain barrier across these neurons helps facilitate glucose sensing. These neurons are classified as glucose-excited (GE) or glucose-inhibited (GI) neurons [45]. Also, peripheral sensory neurons innervating different organs are said to possess glucose sensing mechanisms.

Based on hypo-/hyper-glycaemia, ANS can initiate compensatory responses by altering the insulin-glucagon balance.

### 10.3.4 The Interplay Between ANS and Stress

Stress is any change in internal and/or external environment that can lead to perturbations in homeostasis. The physiological response to stress consists of activation of the neuroendocrine axis leading to promotion of survival responses in the organism. These include two key systems—sympatho-excitation and parasympathetic withdrawal via ANS and release of corticotropin releasing hormone (CRH) by the paraventricular nucleus of the hypothalamus. CRH stimulates the release of adrenocorticotrophic hormone (ACTH), leading to release of glucocorticoids by the adrenal gland. Glucocorticoids are the key effectors of the stress homeostatic response.

Two important cortical areas—medial prefrontal cortex (mPFC) and insular cortex (IC)—help process the physiological responses to stress [48]. mPFC helps inhibit the heart rate response to pathological stress; IC is also implicated in altering cardiac autonomic activity in response to stress.

Paraventricular nucleus (PVN) of the hypothalamus acts as the key integrator of stress response. It receives inputs from various limbic, infralimbic, and other cortical areas. Also, it receives inputs from multiple hypothalamic nuclei such as lateral hypothalamic area, dorso-medial hypothalamus, and posterior hypothalamic areas. PVN projects to brainstem nuclei of ANS regulating cardiovascular responses to stress. In addition, it facilitates releases of glucocorticoids via CRH-mediated ACTH signalling and also causes release of other hormones (Fig. 10.2).

### 10.3.5 The Role of ANS in Appetite and Obesity

ANS also acts as a key regulator of energy balance in our body. It is positioned at a unique place in physiological systems as it can regulate both the food intake and energy expenditure, thereby having an important impact on net body weight.

In the short term, ANS can regulate body weight by control of satiety signals. Satiety is a physiological signal that helps in regulation of the amount of meal being taken by an organism. It is brought about gastric distension following meals and through gastrointestinal hormones [49]. Gastric distension after meals leads to the stimulation of stretch receptors located in the stomach and GI wall due to

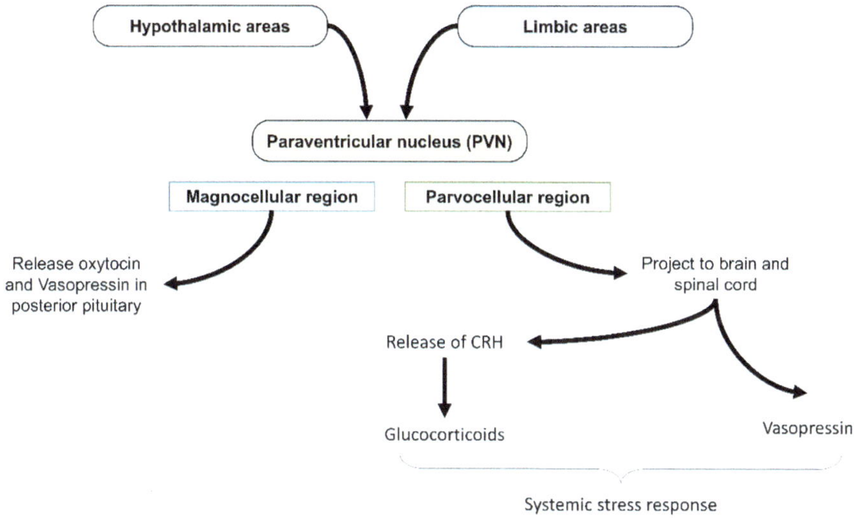


**Fig. 10.2** Paraventricular area as the central integrator of stress

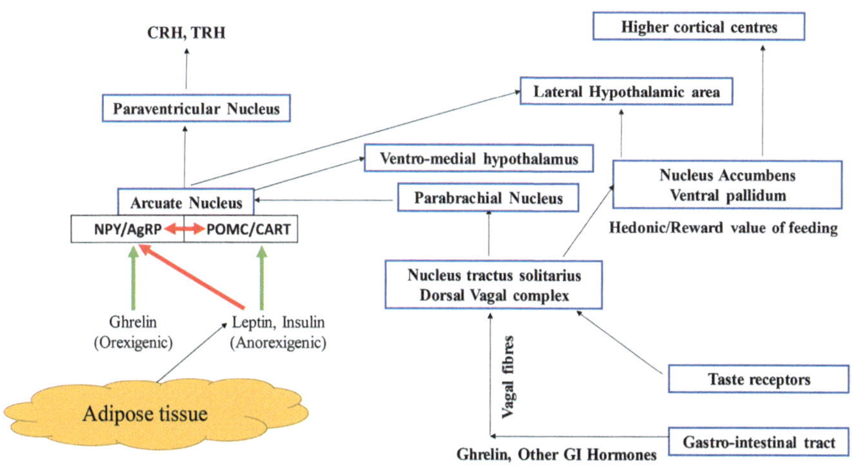


**Fig. 10.3** Regulation of appetite and satiety. Satiety and appetite are based on the interplay between orexigenic and anorexigenic signals acting on different hypothalamic areas. *NPY* neuropeptide Y, *AgRP* agouti related peptide, *POMC* pro-opiomelanocortin, *CART* cocaine- and amphetamine-regulated transcript. (Figure based on information provided in Refs. [50–53])

mechanical stimulation. This stimulus leads to reduction in gastrointestinal motility by short vago-vagal loops. In addition, afferent information is also relayed to the CNS by vagal afferents. Here the signals go directly to the key areas regulating appetite and satiety. The key areas and factors responsible for the balance between appetite and satiety are shown in Fig. 10.3.

ANS also regulates the release of GI hormones that can affect gastric emptying and satiety. These hormones include cholecystokinin, glucagon-like peptide 1, ghrelin, and peptide YY. These peptides act on multiple areas in the hypothalamus to promote the feeling of satiety.

In the long term, ANS regulates energy balance thereby regulating net body weight. This is brought about by leptin, an important adipokine released by adipose tissue stores in the body. Leptin is a 16 kDa peptide hormone released by adipose tissue, though small quantities have also been isolated from the stomach, intestine, muscles, and placenta (137). The peptide was discovered during the attempt at understanding the genetic basis of obesity in mice. Five genes were found to be responsible for obesity—ob gene (encoding for leptin), db gene (responsible for diabetes), agouti yellow, tubby, and fat genes [54, 55]. Leptin is released by white adipose tissue (WAT) and acts to bring about lack of appetite. Leptin levels are shown to increase after feeding and decrease after a bout of fasting, demonstrating its close association with energy balance. This occurs by the action of POMC/CART neurons in the arcuate nucleus while inhibiting NPY/AgRP neurons [56, 57]. This action brings about anorexia and is associated with decreased food intake. Leptin also stimulates lipolysis, thereby promoting energy expenditure. Herein free fatty acids are oxidized to produce energy and create a negative energy balance. In addition, leptin also promotes non-shivering thermogenesis in Brown adipose tissue (BAT) [58].

Thus, the ANS is closely associated with nutrient intake (by acting on the gastrointestinal system), regulation of appetite and satiety, and energy expenditure via SNS. Hence it is an important influence in regulation of body weight.

To summarize, the ANS can act as an important regulator of neuroendocrine system by its structural and neurohumoral connections with the hypothalamus. Elaborate roles of ANS acting as a mediator have been documented in energy balance, glucose homeostasis, and stress.

## References

1. Green JD, Harris GW. The neurovascular link between the neurohypophysis and adenohypophysis. J Endocrinol. 1947;5:136–46.
2. Green JD, Harris GW. Observation of the hypophysio-portal vessels of the living rat. J Physiol. 1949;108:359–61.
3. Harris GW. Neural control of the pituitary gland. Physiol Rev. 1948;28:139–79.
4. Harris GW. The hypothalamus and endocrine glands. Br Med Bull. 1950;6:345–50.
5. Harris GW. Regeneration of the hypophysial portal vessels. Nature. 1948;162:70.
6. Watts AG. The structure of the neuroendocrine hypothalamus: the neuroanatomical legacy of Geoffrey Harris. J Endocrinol. 2015;226:T25–39.
7. Raisman G. 60 Years of Neuroendocrinology: Memoir: Geoffrey Harris and my brush with his unit. J Endocrinol. 2015;226:T1–T11.
8. Silver R, Yao Y, Roy RK, Stern JE. Parallel trajectories in the discovery of the SCN-OVLT and pituitary portal pathways: legacies of Geoffrey Harris. J Neuroendocrinol. 2023;35:e13245.

9. Shahid Z, Asuka E, Singh G. Physiology, hypothalamus. In: StatPearls. Treasure Island: StatPearls Publishing; 2025. http://www.ncbi.nlm.nih.gov/books/NBK535380/. Accessed 13 Nov 2025.
10. Anatomy and function of the hypothalamus | IntechOpen. https://www.intechopen.com/chapters/63258. Accessed 29 Aug 2025.
11. Bear MH, Reddy V, Bollu PC. Neuroanatomy, Hypothalamus. In: StatPearls. Treasure Island: StatPearls Publishing; 2025. http://www.ncbi.nlm.nih.gov/books/NBK525993/. Accessed 13 Nov 2025.
12. Olarescu NC, Gunawardane K, Hanson TK, Møller N, Jørgensen JOL. Normal physiology of growth hormone in normal adults. In: Feingold KR, Ahmed SF, Anawalt B, Blackman MR, Boyce A, Chrousos G, et al., editors. Endotext. South Dartmouth: MDText.com, Inc.; 2000. http://www.ncbi.nlm.nih.gov/books/NBK279056/. Accessed 13 Nov 2025.
13. Granata R. Peripheral activities of growth hormone-releasing hormone. J Endocrinol Invest. 2016;39:721–7.
14. Marques P, De Sousa Lages A, Skorupskaite K, Rozario KS, Anderson RA, George JT. Physiology of GnRH and gonadotrophin secretion. In: Feingold KR, Ahmed SF, Anawalt B, Blackman MR, Boyce A, Chrousos G, et al., editors. Endotext. South Dartmouth: MDText.com, Inc.; 2000. http://www.ncbi.nlm.nih.gov/books/NBK279070/. Accessed 13 Nov 2025.
15. Trevisan CM, Montagna E, de Oliveira R, Christofolini DM, Barbosa CP, Crandall KA, et al. Kisspeptin/GPR54 system: what do we know about its role in human reproduction? Cell Physiol Biochem Int J Exp Cell Physiol Biochem Pharmacol. 2018;49:1259–76.
16. Topaloglu AK, Reimann F, Guclu M, Yalin AS, Kotan LD, Porter KM, et al. TAC3 and TACR3 mutations in familial hypogonadotropic hypogonadism reveal a key role for neurokinin B in the central control of reproduction. Nat Genet. 2009;41:354–8.
17. Goodman RL, Lehman MN, Smith JT, Coolen LM, de Oliveira CVR, Jafarzadehshirazi MR, et al. Kisspeptin neurons in the arcuate nucleus of the ewe express both dynorphin A and neurokinin B. Endocrinology. 2007;148:5752–60.
18. Wang P, Wang SC, Liu X, Jia S, Wang X, Li T, et al. Neural functions of hypothalamic oxytocin and its regulation. ASN Neuro. 2022;14:17590914221100706.
19. Wu G, Ou Y, Feng Z, Xiong Z, Li K, Che M, et al. Oxytocin attenuates hypothalamic injury-induced cognitive dysfunction by inhibiting hippocampal ERK signaling and Aβ deposition. Transl Psychiatry. 2024;14:208.
20. Baribeau DA, Anagnostou E. Oxytocin and vasopressin: linking pituitary neuropeptides and their receptors to social neurocircuits. Front Neurosci. 2015;9:335.
21. Cuzzo B, Padala SA, Lappin SL. Physiology, vasopressin. In: StatPearls. Treasure Island: StatPearls Publishing; 2025. http://www.ncbi.nlm.nih.gov/books/NBK526069/. Accessed 30 Aug 2025.
22. Zimmerman EA, Robinson AG. Hypothalamic neurons secreting vasopressin and neurophysin. Kidney Int. 1976;10:12–24.
23. Trubacova R, Drastichova Z, Novotny J. Biochemical and physiological insights into TRH receptor-mediated signaling. Front Cell Dev Biol. 2022;10. https://doi.org/10.3389/fcell.2022.981452.
24. Hollowell JG, Staehling NW, Dana Flanders W, Harry Hannon W, Gunter EW, Spencer CA, et al. Serum TSH, T4, and thyroid antibodies in the United States population (1988 to 1994): National Health and Nutrition Examination Survey (NHANES III). J Clin Endocrinol Metab. 2002;87:489–99.
25. Choi Y-H, Hartzell D, Azain MJ, Baile CA. TRH decreases food intake and increases water intake and body temperature in rats. Physiol Behav. 2002;77:1–4.
26. Tsuru J, Ishitobi Y, Ninomiya T, Kanehisa M, Imanaga J, Inoue A, et al. The thyrotropin-releasing hormone test may predict recurrence of clinical depression within ten years after discharge. Neuro Endocrinol Lett. 2013;34:409–17.
27. Shibusawa N, Hashimoto K, Yamada M. Thyrotropin-releasing hormone (TRH) in the cerebellum. Cerebellum Lond Engl. 2008;7:84–95.

28. Caruso A, Gaetano A, Scaccianoce S. Corticotropin-releasing hormone: biology and therapeutic opportunities. Biology. 2022;11:1785.
29. McLean M, Smith R. Corticotrophin-releasing hormone and human parturition. 2001. https://doi.org/10.1530/rep.0.1210493.
30. Smith R, Nicholson RC. Corticotrophin releasing hormone and the timing of birth. Front Biosci J Virtual Libr. 2007;12:912–8.
31. Nezi M, Mastorakos G, Mouslech Z. Corticotropin releasing hormone and the immune/inflammatory response. In: Feingold KR, Ahmed SF, Anawalt B, Blackman MR, Boyce A, Chrousos G, et al., editors. Endotext. South Dartmouth: MDText.com, Inc.; 2000. http://www.ncbi.nlm.nih.gov/books/NBK279017/. Accessed 12 Nov 2025.
32. Stagkourakis S, Kim H, Lyons DJ, Broberger C. Dopamine autoreceptor regulation of a hypothalamic dopaminergic network. Cell Rep. 2016;15:735.
33. Osilla EV, Marsidi JL, Shumway KR, Sharma S. Physiology, temperature regulation. In: StatPearls. Treasure Island: StatPearls Publishing; 2025. http://www.ncbi.nlm.nih.gov/books/NBK507838/. Accessed 13 Nov 2025.
34. Miller JB. Hyperthermia and fever. In: Silverstein DC, Hopper K, editors. Small animal critical care medicine. Elsevier Saunders, Philadelphia; 2009. p. 21–26.
35. Abizaid A, Horvath TL. Ghrelin and the central regulation of feeding and energy balance. Indian J Endocrinol Metab. 2012;16:S617–26.
36. Ma MA, Morrison EH. Neuroanatomy, nucleus suprachiasmatic. In: StatPearls. Treasure Island: StatPearls Publishing; 2025. http://www.ncbi.nlm.nih.gov/books/NBK546664/. Accessed 13 Nov 2025.
37. Saper CB, Lowell BB. The hypothalamus. Curr Biol. 2014;24:R1111–6.
38. Kaur M, Srivastav S, Jaryal AK, Deepak KK. Baroreflex dysfunction in Prader Willi syndrome. J Clin Diagn Res JCDR. 2016;10:CD01–2.
39. Mishra A, Sharma R, Mittal P, Kapoor R, Srivastav S. Evaluating exercise challenge to validate cardiac autonomic dysfunction in lean PCOS phenotype. J Basic Clin Physiol Pharmacol. 2019;30. https://doi.org/10.1515/jbcpp-2018-0198.
40. Ravichandran S, Srivastav S, Kamble PH, Chambial S, Shukla R, Sharma P, et al. VEGF-A and cardiac autonomic function in newly diagnosed type 2 diabetes mellitus: a cross-sectional study at a tertiary care center. J Fam Med Prim Care. 2019;8:3185–90.
41. Shobhawat M, Srivastav S, Shukla RG, Bhagat OL. Assessing the Impact of BMI and Glycaemic Control on Cardiac Autonomic Neuropathy in Patients with Early and Long-standing Diabetes Mellitus: A Window of Opportunity. Ann Neurosci. 2025 Nov 21:09727531251384548. https://doi.org/10.1177/09727531251384548. Epub ahead of print. PMID: 41280749; PMCID: PMC12638237.
42. Oakes PC, Fisahn C, Iwanaga J, DiLorenzo D, Oskouian RJ, Tubbs RS. A history of the autonomic nervous system: part I: from Galen to Bichat. Childs Nerv Syst ChNS Off J Int Soc Pediatr Neurosurg. 2016;32:2303–8.
43. Oakes PC, Fisahn C, Iwanaga J, DiLorenzo D, Oskouian RJ, Tubbs RS. A history of the autonomic nervous system: part II: from Reil to the modern era. Childs Nerv Syst ChNS Off J Int Soc Pediatr Neurosurg. 2016;32:2309–15.
44. Lemery R. The autonomic nervous system and the origins of neurocardiology. J Cardiovasc Electrophysiol. 2024;35:1665–72.
45. Faber CL, Deem JD, Campos CA, Taborsky GJ, Morton GJ. CNS control of the endocrine pancreas. Diabetologia. 2020;63:2086–94.
46. Tang S-C, Baeyens L, Shen C-N, Peng S-J, Chien H-J, Scheel DW, et al. Human pancreatic neuro-insular network in health and fatty infiltration. Diabetologia. 2018;61:168–81.
47. Thorens B. Neuronal glucose sensing mechanisms and circuits in the control of insulin and glucagon secretion. Physiol Rev. 2024;104:1461–86.
48. Schaeuble D, Myers B. Cortical-hypothalamic integration of autonomic and endocrine stress responses. Front Physiol. 2022;13:820398.
49. Guarino D, Nannipieri M, Iervasi G, Taddei S, Bruno RM. The role of the autonomic nervous system in the pathophysiology of obesity. Front Physiol. 2017;8:665.

50. Kojima M, Hosoda H, Date Y, Nakazato M, Matsuo H, Kangawa K. Ghrelin is a growth-hormone-releasing acylated peptide from stomach. Nature. 1999;402:656–60.
51. Saper CB, Chou TC, Elmquist JK. The need to feed: homeostatic and hedonic control of eating. Neuron. 2002;36:199–211.
52. Morton GJ, Cummings DE, Baskin DG, Barsh GS, Schwartz MW. Central nervous system control of food intake and body weight. Nature. 2006;443:289–95.
53. Cummings DE. Ghrelin and the short- and long-term regulation of appetite and body weight. Physiol Behav. 2006;89:71–84.
54. Scharf MT, Ahima RS. Gut peptides and other regulators in obesity. Semin Liver Dis. 2004;24:335–47.
55. Gurevich-Panigrahi T, Panigrahi S, Wiechec E, Los M. Obesity: pathophysiology and clinical management. Curr Med Chem. 2009;16:506–21.
56. Bodur C, Duensing A, Myers MG. Molecular mechanisms and neural mediators of leptin action. Genes Dev. 2025;39:792–807.
57. Myers MG, Cowley MA, Münzberg H. Mechanisms of leptin action and leptin resistance. Annu Rev Physiol. 2008;70:537–56.
58. Seoane-Collazo P, Martínez-Sánchez N, Milbank E, Contreras C. Incendiary leptin. Nutrients. 2020:12. https://doi.org/10.3390/nu12020472.

# Hypophysiotropic Neuroendocrine Axes and Neuroendocrine Regulation

11

Bhawna Mattoo

**Abstract**

Hypophysiotropic neuroendocrine axes represent the primary regulatory pathways through which the hypothalamus integrates neural and hormonal signals to maintain homeostasis. This chapter outlines the organization and regulation of the major hypothalamic–pituitary axes, including the adrenal, thyroid, gonadal, somatotropic, and lactotropic axes. The roles of hypothalamic-releasing and inhibitory hormones, pituitary tropic hormones, and peripheral endocrine glands are described, with emphasis on feedback control, pulsatile secretion, and circadian regulation. Unique features of individual axes, as well as direct hypothalamic control of posterior pituitary hormones, are briefly reviewed, highlighting their physiological and clinical relevance.

**Keywords**

Hypothalamus · Pituitary gland · Hypothalamic–pituitary axis · Neuroendocrine regulation · Feedback control · Hormonal rhythms

## 11.1 Introduction

Within the hypothalamus lies the body's homeostatic thermostat. Many physiological functions, including metabolism, growth, stress responses, osmoregulation, and circadian rhythm, are regulated by it. The neuroendocrine axis is a three-tier regulatory system. The top tier is at the level of the hypothalamus. The middle one is at the level of the pituitary, and the bottom is at the level of the target organs. There are five major neuroendocrine (hypothalamic–pituitary) axes, each organized around a hypothalamic-releasing hormone, a pituitary tropic hormone, and a peripheral target organ: hypothalamic–pituitary–adrenal (HPA) axis,

B. Mattoo (✉)
ESIC Medical College and Hospital, Faridabad, Haryana, India





H. Prabhakar, M. Kaur (eds.), *Brain and Endocrine Crosstalk*, Physiology in Clinical Neurosciences – Brain and Spinal Cord Crosstalks,
https://doi.org/10.1007/978-981-92-0763-3_11

hypothalamic–pituitary–thyroid (HPT) axis, hypothalamic–pituitary–gonadal (HPG) axis, hypothalamic–pituitary–somatotropic (HPS) axis, and the hypothalamic–pituitary–lactotropic (HPL) axis.

Endocrine functions of the pituitary gland are regulated by the hypothalamus and by negative and positive feedback loops within this three-tier system. Several cells in the hypothalamus are neuroendocrine, releasing their neurotransmitter into the bloodstream. The hypothalamic neuroendocrine cells regulate both the anterior and posterior pituitary by releasing stimulatory or inhibitory factors. A region within the hypothalamus known as the hypophysiotropic area contains groups of small (parvocellular) neurons whose axons extend to the median eminence. The releasing hormones first enter a primary network of fenestrated capillaries and are transported via the Hypothalamic-pituitary adrenal axis but here it will be hypothalamo-hypophyseal portal system—which connect one capillary bed to another without passing through the heart—to a secondary capillary plexus in the pars distalis. The large magnocellular cells of the paraventricular nucleus (PVN) and supraoptic nucleus (SON) send their projections to the posterior pituitary (pars nervosa) directly [3].

Each endocrine axis operates around an individualized set point. This is regulated primarily by negative feedback from the peripheral hormone itself and not by the physiological effects of the hormone. When hormone levels fall, hypothalamic and pituitary output rise, and when hormone levels rise, they suppress further release. Because the feedback loop depends mainly on the hormone—not on every organ it influences—each axis functions semi-independently. This allows each hormone to affect multiple systems without those systems directly regulating the hormone.

Most of these hormones have a rhythm to their secretion, which is entrained to various biological cues. Their pulsatility may have ultradian, or seasonal rhythms. The hypothalamus does not work in isolation and receives many neural signals from different parts of the brain—some temporary (like stress or illness) and some long-lasting (like the developmental changes that occur at puberty), and because the hypothalamus is part of each endocrine axis, it can combine all this information and adjust the axis's set point accordingly. In other words, the hypothalamus serves as a central integrator that allows endocrine systems to adapt to both short-term and long-term physiological demands.

## 11.2 Hypothalamic–Pituitary–Adrenal (HPA) Axis

The HPA axis is also known as the stress axis as it is pivotal in our response to stress. It provides a neuroendocrine mechanism which mediates the effects of stressors by regulating numerous physiological processes, such as metabolism, immune responses, and the autonomic responses. At the top of this axis is the hypothalamic corticotropin-releasing hormone (CRH), produced majorly in the medial parvocellular part of the PVN. CRH is a 41-amino-acid peptide released into the portal vasculature, where it targets the corticotropes of the anterior pituitary gland. The magnocellular neurons release arginine vasopressin (AVP), another hypothalamic hormone which acts at pituitary corticotropes to exert synergistic effects. The corticotropes have receptors for and respond to both CRH and AVP to cause the release of adrenocorticotropic hormone (ACTH) from the corticotropes. Once ACTH is in the systemic circulation, it acts at receptors on the adrenal cortex to stimulate the production and release of glucocorticoids. The glucocorticoids have negative feedback on the brain and pituitary (Fig. 11.1).

At the anterior pituitary, cortisol binds to cytosolic glucocorticoid receptors in corticotropes. The hormone–receptor complex translocates to the nucleus, binds to glucocorticoid response elements (GREs), and modulates gene expression. This inhibits the synthesis of the CRH receptor and ACTH, primarily by suppressing transcription of the proopiomelanocortin (*POMC*) gene. Cortisol also inhibits the release of stored ACTH granules. At the hypothalamus, cortisol reduces both the mRNA and peptide levels of CRH in PVN neurons. It also inhibits the secretion of preformed CRH. Although present, hypothalamic feedback is less dominant than feedback at the pituitary. Chronic ACTH elevation (e.g., chronic stress) causes adrenal hypertrophy, high glucocorticoid levels, and sometimes adrenal exhaustion [12].

ACTH has minimal effect on aldosterone. Its primary regulators are potassium, sodium, blood volume, and angiotensin II. Adrenalectomy lowers liver glycogen and blood glucose due to reduced gluconeogenesis. Cortisol increases blood glucose by decreasing glucose use and increasing gluconeogenesis. Glucagon raises blood glucose, whereas insulin lowers it and promotes glycogen storage. Stress elevates CRH → ACTH → glucocorticoids. Responses may be brief or chronic. Glucocorticoids raise circulating glucose but, when elevated long term, suppress

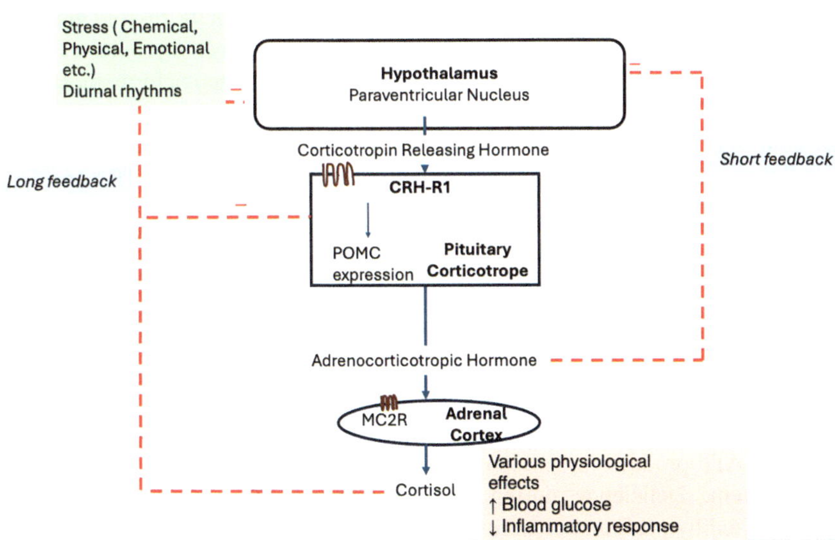


**Fig. 11.1** depicts the hypothalamic–pituitary–adrenal axis. *CRH-R1* corticotropin-releasing hormone, *ACTH* adrenocorticotropic hormone, *MC2R* melanocortin-2 receptor, *POMC* proopiomelanocortin

reproduction (at hypothalamus, pituitary, and gonads) and depress immune function.Glucocorticoids also induce apoptosis in developing immune cells (autoreactive T and B cells) and, when chronically high, can cause immune suppression in adults by promoting apoptosis of immune cells [7]. Aldosterone maintains salt balance by promoting renal $Na^+$ reabsorption. Lack of aldosterone (e.g., after adrenalectomy) rapidly causes $Na^+$ loss and circulatory collapse unless $Na^+$ or aldosterone is replaced.

Stress-related hormones are released in both pulsatile bursts and daily (circadian) cycles. If the suprachiasmatic nucleus (SCN)—the brain's circadian pacemaker—is damaged, the normal 24-h rhythm of CRH secretion disappears [11]. In humans, glucocorticoid concentrations are highest in the early morning (around 07:00) and lowest in the afternoon. HPA axis dysregulation is a significant covariate for various subgroups of disorders, and it has been associated with differential treatment responsiveness, recovery rate, and probability of disease relapse [10].

## 11.3 Hypothalamic–Pituitary–Thyroid (HPT) Axis

The thyrotropic axis primarily regulates cellular metabolism and organismal development. At the top of this axis is the thyrotropin-releasing hormone (TRH), synthesized by neurons in the parvocellular division of the paraventricular nucleus (PVN) of the hypothalamus. These neurons project to the median eminence and release TRH into the hypophysial portal system, which delivers it to the anterior pituitary. TRH acts on thyrotrope cells in the anterior pituitary—making up about 10% of its cell population—to promote the secretion of thyroid-stimulating hormone (TSH). Once released into the bloodstream, TSH binds to receptors in the thyroid gland and stimulates the production and release of the thyroid hormones thyroxine (T4) and triiodothyronine (T3). Although T3 is the more biologically active form, most of the hormone produced and circulating is T4, which is subsequently converted to T3 in the brain, pituitary, brown fat, and other peripheral tissues by type I and type II deiodinase enzymes. T3 acts on nuclear thyroid hormone receptors (TRα and TRβ) located throughout the body, including brain, autonomic nervous system, pituitary, muscle, bone, and liver, highlighting its systemic importance. These receptors function as transcription factors, typically forming heterodimers with Retinoid X Receptor (RXR) to regulate gene expression. In the hypothalamus and pituitary, thyroid hormones exert classic negative feedback: they inhibit TRH release from PVN neurons and suppress TSH synthesis in thyrotropes, thereby maintaining stable circulating hormone levels (Fig. 11.2).

Thyroid hormone is essential for basal metabolic rate, protein synthesis, mitochondrial ATP production, and normal development, especially of the central nervous system. Deficiency during fetal or neonatal life results in cretinism, characterized by profound cognitive and physical impairments, which can be prevented with timely newborn screening and replacement therapy. TRH and TSH are released in a pulsatile manner, with TSH demonstrating a circadian rhythm driven by the suprachiasmatic nucleus. TSH levels peak during the night (the "nocturnal

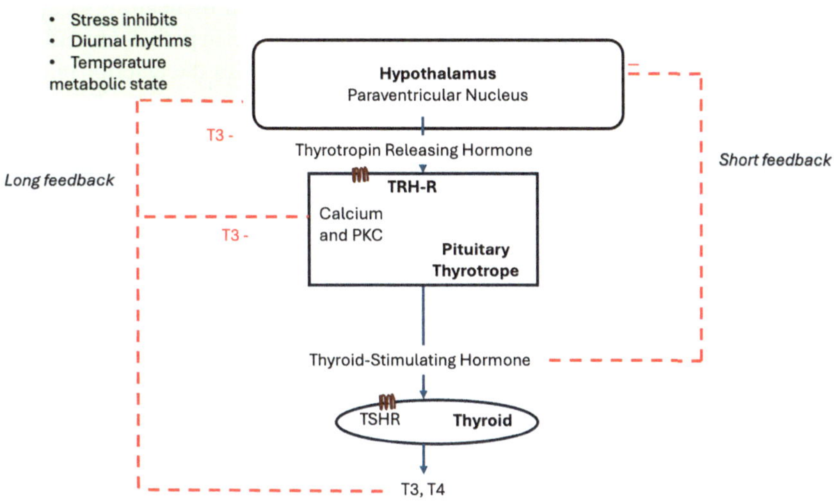


**Fig. 11.2** Hypothalamic–pituitary–thyroid axis. *PKA* protein kinase A, *PKC* protein kinase C, *T3* triiodothyronine (active form of thyroid hormone), *T4* thyroxine, *TRH* thyrotropin-releasing hormone, *TSH* thyroid-stimulating hormone

TSH surge") and decline toward midday. The diurnal TSH rhythm is independent of the negative feedback mechanism.

The hypothalamus regulates the hypothalamic–pituitary–thyroid axis largely via incoming neural signals from two functionally opposing neuronal groups within the arcuate nucleus. One group consists of proopiomelanocortin (POMC) neurons, which also express cocaine- and amphetamine-regulated transcript (CART), while the other comprises neuropeptide-Y (NPY) neurons that co-express agouti-related peptides. Although distinct, both populations possess receptors for leptin, an adipocyte-derived hormone [1].

Alpha-melanocyte-stimulating hormone (α-MSH) and CART stimulate transcription of the *TRH* gene in hypophysiotropic neurons, whereas NPY and agouti-related peptide exert an inhibitory influence [8]. As a result, when leptin levels fall during fasting, the sensitivity of hypophysiotropic TRH neurons to thyroid hormone feedback increases, effectively reducing TRH output [8].

This regulatory mechanism is evolutionarily conserved and has been observed across multiple animal species, including humans.

## 11.4 Hypothalamic–Pituitary–Gonadal (HPG) Axis

Gonadal function is shaped by interactions across three levels: central: hypothalamus and anterior pituitary; intermediate: gonadal tissue and circulating hormones; and peripheral: target organs responding to sex steroids.

Gonadotropin-releasing hormone (GnRH) is synthesized by neurons located in the preoptic area, anterior hypothalamus, and medio-basal hypothalamus. This is released in the hypophyseal portal circulation and stimulates the anterior pituitary to release LH and FSH. These gonadotropins drive steroid hormone production and gamete formation in the gonads. An increase in gonadal steroids exerts negative feedback on both hypothalamic and pituitary centers, while gonadal peptides such as inhibin and activin modulate gonadotropin synthesis primarily at the pituitary level. Feedback regulation operates through long-loop pathways (gonads → hypothalamus), short-loop pathways (gonads → pituitary), and ultrashort-loop control within the gonads themselves (Fig. 11.3).

GnRH release is characteristically pulsatile (~one pulse/hour) and, in females, includes a large preovulatory surge. Tonic pulsatility is governed mainly by steroid-sensitive circuits in the medial basal hypothalamus, whereas the additional inputs required for the ovulatory surge require additional inputs. Steroid hormones also directly influence pituitary gonadotropes by regulating GnRH receptor expression, cell proliferation, and gonadotropin gene transcription, alongside direct actions on steroidogenic cells. In spontaneous ovulators such as humans, progressively rising estradiol (E2) from maturing follicles heightens pituitary sensitivity to GnRH and eventually switches feedback to positive, triggering the GnRH/LH surge responsible for ovulation and corpus luteum formation. After ovulation, E2 and progesterone support endometrial growth and readiness for implantation, and withdrawal of these hormones initiates menstruation and a new cycle. E2 exerts biphasic feedback: Low–moderate levels suppress LH and FSH, while high preovulatory levels induce positive feedback and the LH surge. Progesterone initially enhances GnRH signaling but later imposes strong negative feedback to prevent additional cycles. Together, E2 and

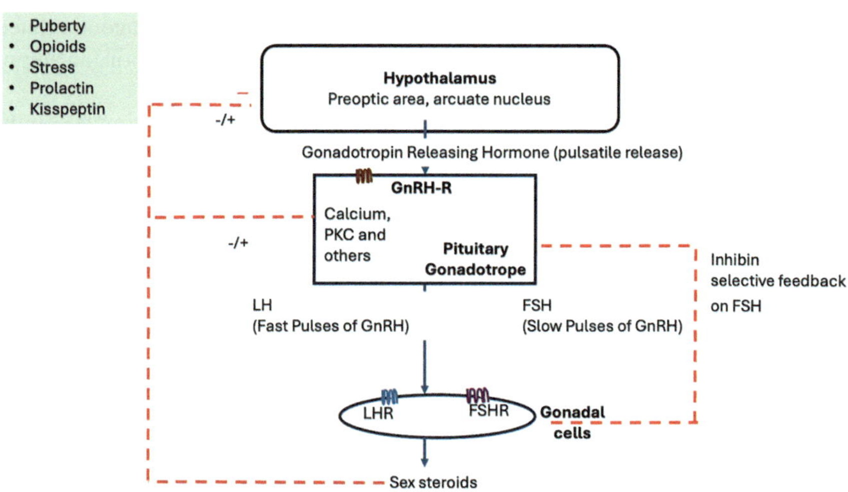


**Fig. 11.3** Hypothalamic–pituitary–gonadal axis. *FSH* follicle-stimulating hormone, *GnRH* gonadotropin-releasing hormone, *GnRH-R* gonadotropin-releasing hormone receptor, *LH* luteinizing hormone, *FSHR* follicle-stimulating hormone receptor, *LHR* luteinizing hormone receptor

progesterone regulate the uterus, cervix, and mammary tissue and influence sexual receptivity in many species. Puberty is characterized by increased GnRH pulsatility, followed by rises in LH and FSH [13]. In girls, this initiates follicular activity, breast development, growth acceleration, and ultimately menarche [4]. In males, GnRH pulses are slower and do not exhibit surges. LH stimulates testosterone synthesis by Leydig cells, while FSH supports Sertoli cell function and spermatogenesis. Testosterone feeds back to both hypothalamus and pituitary either directly as an androgen or after conversion to estradiol. Because GnRH neurons express minimal receptors for E2 or androgens, feedback appears to act indirectly via interneurons.

Androgens maintain spermatogenesis, male sexual behaviors, and accessory gland activity. Conversion of testosterone to DHT drives growth and secretory function of the prostate and seminal vesicles. Continuous androgen exposure is necessary for normal adult male reproductive physiology.

Developmentally four stages are recognized in the gonadal axis: fetal, perinatal, prepubertal, and pubertal. Testosterone secretion begins around week 8 under placental gonadotropin control, while pituitary gonadotropins appear by the 12th week. After birth, HPG activity drives transient testicular and likely ovarian hormone production in the initial 6 months of life. Before puberty, gonadostat sensitivity to steroids is high, suppressing gonadotropins to minimal levels, and at the onset of puberty, the threshold resets upward; LH/FSH pulses increase, triggering secondary sexual development and fertility. Large nocturnal LH–testosterone bursts and positive estrogen feedback enabling ovulation appear.

The discovery of kisspeptin transformed the understanding of reproductive neuroendocrine regulation. Kisspeptin binding to its receptor (KISS1R) activates GnRH secretion and thereby drives the HPG axis. Neurons in the arcuate nucleus expressing kisspeptin, neurokinin B, and dynorphin—known as KNDy neurons—mediate both positive and negative estrogen feedback on GnRH release. Kisspeptin is crucial for puberty onset and regulates follicle growth, oocyte maturation, and ovulation [6]. In males, it supports Leydig cell function, spermatogenesis, sperm physiology, and reproductive behavior. Disturbances in kisspeptin/KISS1R signaling can lead to conditions such as idiopathic hypogonadotropic hypogonadism (iHH), central precocious puberty (CPP), and infertility. Insights into kisspeptin pathways may guide future therapeutic strategies.

## 11.5 Hypothalamic–Pituitary–Somatotropic (HPS) Axis

Growth and metabolism are closely regulated by the somatotropic axis. Its distinctive feature lies at the top tier of regulation wherein a delicate balance between two kinds of hypothalamic factors, the growth hormone–releasing factor (GHRH) and somatostatin, decides the directional swing of the axis. GHRH promotes growth hormone (GH) secretion, and somatostatin inhibits it. GH, or somatotropin, is released from specialized cells in the anterior pituitary gland called somatotropes. which form around 30 % of the anterior pituitary cell) (Fig. 11.4).

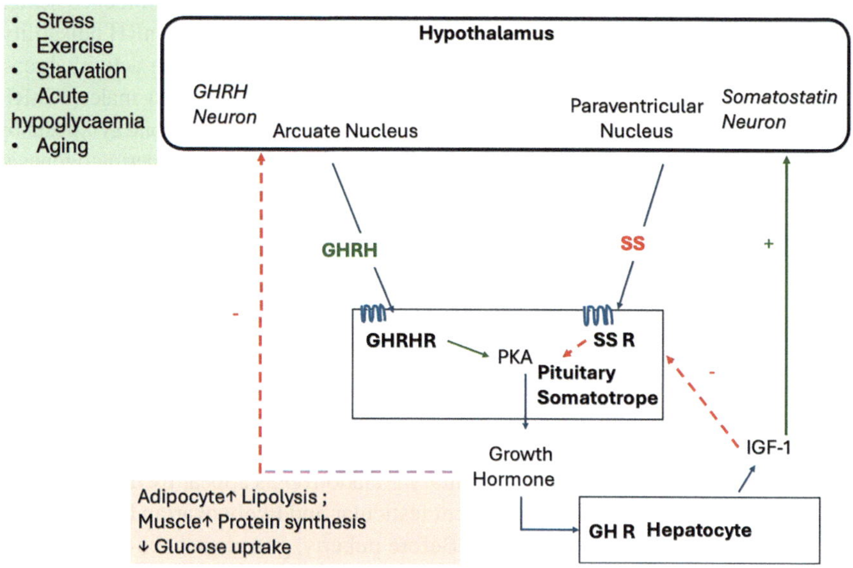


**Fig. 11.4** Hypothalamic–pituitary–somatotropic axis. *GHRH* growth hormone–releasing hormone, *GHRHR* growth hormone–releasing hormone receptor, *IGF-I* insulin-like growth factor I, *SS* somatostatin, *SS R* somatostatin receptor

GH stimulates the liver and other tissues to produce insulin-like growth factor I (IGF-I). Together, GH and IGF-I support tissue growth, protein synthesis, lipid breakdown, carbohydrate metabolism, and overall metabolic balance.

They also operate within intricate feedback loops—GH and IGF-I dampen GHRH release while increasing somatostatin production—to maintain precise control of growth and metabolic signaling.

GHRH neurons are localized within the arcuate nucleus of the hypothalamus, while somatostatin is formed in the periventricular nucleus of the anterior hypothalamus.

Both these hormones are released in the portal capillary vasculature, causing the release of GH by the somatotropes. GH further binds to its receptors on the liver to release IGF-I. Both GH and IGF-1 are important in the feedback regulation seen in the somatotropic axis. They give a negative feedback and cause downregulation of GHRH, while it stimulates gene expression of somatostatin. Vasoactive intestinal peptide, dopamine, TRH, pituitary adenylate cyclase–activating peptide, galanin, neuropeptide Y, motilin, and interleukins also play a role in the regulation of the somatotropic axis. As growth is a highly integrated activity, inputs from other hormones, such as the thyroid hormone, glucocorticoids, sex steroid hormones, and metabolic fuels, can influence the release of growth. IGF-1 is particularly noted for its growth-promoting effects in the central nervous system. As IGF-I can cross the blood–brain barrier, it can also act as a negative feedback regulator of GHRH neurons. At higher doses, IGF-I can stimulate somatostatin release. In the circulation, it binds to several binding proteins like IGF-I binding protein 3 (IGFBP-3). As free IG 1 is more biologically active, levels of IGFBP-3 are important in deciding the activity of GH.

Both GHRH and somatostatin are released in a pulsatile and coordinated fashion from hypothalamic nerve terminals into the portal circulation. The growth hormone is released in a diurnal pattern being associated with sleep, highest levels after onset of slow-wave sleep, and most GH secretion occurs at night in humans [5].

As we age, the levels of GH also fall, as lower levels of the hormone are released in each burst. It decreases by half every 10 years after the age of 20. This is referred to as "somatopause," and a significant fall in IGF-1 levels is also noted.

## 11.6 Hypothalamic–Pituitary–Prolactin Axis

The lactation axis is unique in that it has no prolactin-releasing hormone. Prolactin is the main hormone for lactation. Dopamine is known to have an inhibitory action over the lactation axis (Fig. 11.5).

It is released by three neuroendocrine dopaminergic neurons: the tuberoinfundibular dopaminergic (TIDA), tuberohypophyseal dopaminergic, and periventricular hypophyseal dopaminergic neurons [2]. The TIDA neurons provide major dopaminergic input to the anterior pituitary. During late pregnancy and lactation, the met-enkephalin released by TIDA neurons can promote the secretion of prolactin. The met-enkephalin also directly enhances the secretory activity of lactotrophs besides

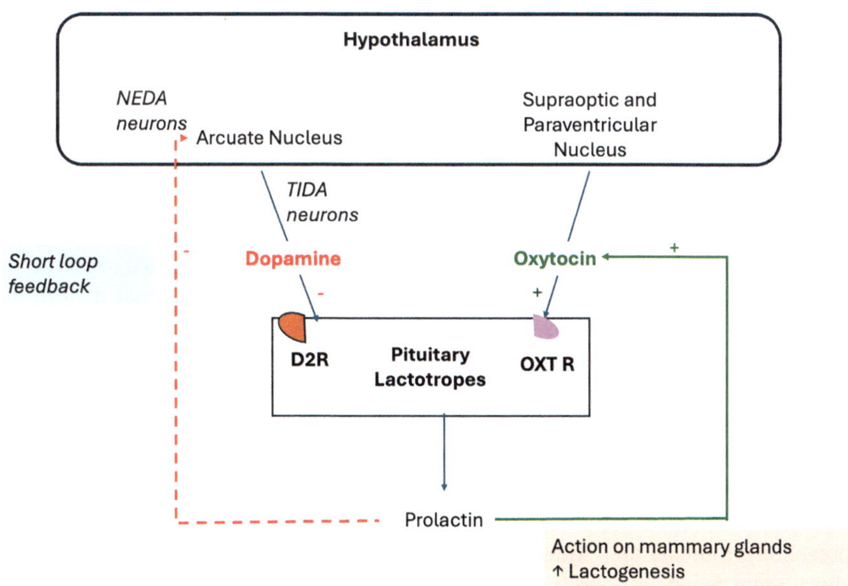


**Fig. 11.5** Hypothalamic–pituitary lactation axis. *NEDA* neuroendocrine dopaminergic neurons, *TIDA* tuberoinfundibular dopaminergic, *D2R* dopamine receptor, *OXT R* oxytocin receptor

traveling through the portal vessels [15]. Dopamine acts on the $D_2$ receptors present on the pituitary lactotropes and decreases the cAMP, which inhibits the gene transcription of dopamine. Oxytocin, a nine-amino acid neuropeptide, recognized for its roles in parturition, uterine contractions, and lactation, stimulates the release of prolactin. It is synthesized in the paraventricular and supraoptic nuclei of the hypothalamus and reaches oxytocin receptors on anterior pituitary lactotrophs via the long and short portal vessels. Prolactin has also been shown to increase neuronal nitric oxide synthase (nNOS) activity within the PVN and SON, thereby influencing the regulation of oxytocin and vasopressin release during the maternal adaptations of late pregnancy and lactation [14]. Suckling is the main stimulus for pituitary lactotropes to release prolactin. Prolactin controls milk ejection, while oxytocin controls milk production. TRH and Vasoactive Intestinal Peptide (VIP) may also stimulate prolactin release. Prolactin levels vary across the sexes and are higher in females than males, being even higher in the luteal phase of the menstrual cycle. It increases during pregnancy, drops before birth, and rises again during suckling. Prolactin plays a crucial role in mammary gland development and lactation. It promotes the growth of ductal and alveolar structures and increases casein mRNA and protein production. Suckling can suppress ovulation and implantation, contributing to lactational infertility. In the ovary, prolactin upregulates LH receptors in the corpus luteum, enhances progesterone synthesis, and influences lipid binding within luteal cells. It may also contribute to maternal behavior. Prolactin release occurs in pulses and follows a sleep-related diurnal pattern rather than an intrinsic circadian rhythm.

## 11.7 Hypothalamic Regulation of the Posterior Pituitary Hormones

While the adenohypophysial system is mediated by the portal capillary vasculature system, the neurohypophysial system is a direct neural link between the hypothalamus and pituitary. This neural innervation of the posterior pituitary enables prompt regulation, set off by changes in blood osmolarity (AVP) or the suckling stimulus (oxytocin), both of which require immediate responses. It thus acts as a neuroendocrine reflex arc. AVP and oxytocin are synthesized in the unmyelinated axons of the magnocellular neurons of the hypothalamus but are stored and released from the posterior pituitary. Unlike the anterior pituitary gland, the posterior pituitary gland does not rely on portal circulation or regulatory hormones from the hypothalamus. It releases hormones directly into the systemic circulation, which are stored as neurosecretory granules in Herring's bodies at the axon terminals. AVP, or antidiuretic hormone (ADH), is synthesized in the supraoptic nuclei of the hypothalamus, whereas oxytocin is synthesized in the paraventricular nuclei of the hypothalamus. Once released into the systemic circulation, they bind to their respective target sites, preventing diuresis and stimulating lactation and/or uterine contraction. It has a short, rapid feedback loop based on plasma osmolarity, blood volume, or sensory input. This is unlike the complex long-loop hormonal feedback in the anterior pituitary.

AVP participates in regulating the stress response, in part, by traveling through the hypophysial portal vessels to act directly on corticotropic cells in the anterior pituitary. Additionally, AVP released from the neurohypophysis influences body fluid osmolality, which can indirectly alter activity within the hypothalamic–pituitary–adrenal axis. Together with oxytocin, AVP is critical in governing social and reproductive behaviors, including parental care and the formation of pair bonds [9]. It is present and conserved across vertebrates, indicating its fundamental survival functions.

## References


1. Ahima RS, Saper CB, Flier JS, Elmquist JK. Leptin regulation of neuroendocrine systems. Front Neuroendocrinol. 2000;21(3):263–307.
2. DeMaria JE, Lerant AA, Freeman ME. Prolactin activates all three populations of hypothalamic neuroendocrine dopaminergic neurons in ovariectomized rats. Brain Res. 1999;837(1–2):236–41. https://doi.org/10.1016/s0006-8993(99)01667-4.
3. Koeppen BM, Stanton BA, Hall JM, Swiatecka-Urban A. Berne & Levy physiology. 8th ed. Elsevier. Springer, Boston, MA. 2024.
4. Gore, A.C. GnRH: The Master Molecule of Reproduction. Elsevier, Philadelphia, PA. 2002.
5. Gore AC. Neuroendocrine targets of endocrine disruptors. Hormones (Athens, Greece). 2010;9(1):16–27. https://doi.org/10.14310/horm.2002.1249.
6. Han SK, Gottsch ML, Lee KJ, Popa SM, Smith JT, Jakawich SK, Clifton DK, Steiner RA, Herbison AE. Activation of gonadotropin-releasing hormone neurons by kisspeptin as a neuroendocrine switch for the onset of puberty. J Neurosci. 2005;25(49):11349–56. https://doi.org/10.1523/JNEUROSCI.3328-05.2005.
7. Herman JP, McKlveen JM, Ghosal S, Kopp B, Wulsin A, Makinson R, Scheimann J, Myers B. Regulation of the hypothalamic-pituitary-adrenocortical stress response. Compr Physiol. 2016;6(2):603–21. https://doi.org/10.1002/cphy.c150015.
8. Lechan RM, Toni R. Functional anatomy of the hypothalamus and pituitary. Endotext [Internet]. 2016.
9. Lim MM, Young LJ. Neuropeptidergic regulation of affiliative behavior and social bonding in animals. Horm Behav. 2006;50(4):506–17. https://doi.org/10.1016/j.yhbeh.2006.06.028.
10. Ring M. An integrative approach to HPA Axis dysfunction: from recognition to recovery. Am J Med. 2025;138(10):1451–63. https://doi.org/10.1016/j.amjmed.2025.05.044.
11. Spencer RL, Deak T. A users guide to HPA axis research. Physiol Behav. 2017;178:43–65. https://doi.org/10.1016/j.physbeh.2016.11.014.
12. Sheng JA, Bales NJ, Myers SA, Bautista AI, Roueinfar M, Hale TM, Handa RJ. The hypothalamic-pituitary-adrenal axis: development, programming actions of hormones, and maternal-fetal interactions. Front Behav Neurosci. 2021;14:601939. https://doi.org/10.3389/fnbeh.2020.601939.
13. Sisk CL, Foster DL. The neural basis of puberty and adolescence. Nat Neurosci. 2004;7:1040–7.
14. Vega C, Moreno-Carranza B, Zamorano M, Quintanar-Stéphano A, Méndez I, Thebault S, Martínez de la Escalera G, Clapp C. Prolactin promotes oxytocin and vasopressin release by activating neuronal nitric oxide synthase in the supraoptic and paraventricular nuclei. Am J Physiol Regul Integr Comp Physiol. 2010;299(6):R1701–8. https://doi.org/10.1152/ajpregu.00575.2010.
15. Yip SH, Romanò N, Gustafson P, Hodson DJ, Williams EJ, Kokay IC, Martin AO, Mollard P, Grattan DR, Bunn SJ. Elevated prolactin during pregnancy drives a phenotypic switch in mouse hypothalamic dopaminergic neurons. Cell Rep. 2019;26(7):1787–1799.e5. https://doi.org/10.1016/j.celrep.2019.01.067.

# Neuroendocrine Adaptations to Physiological and Clinical Conditions

12

Manpreet Kaur

**Abstract**

The neuroendocrine system is a two-way communication between the nervous and endocrine systems, enabling homeostatic regulation across a wide range of physiological and clinical conditions. This enables integration of central neural circuits with peripheral hormonal signals and aids in modulation of vital physiological functions such as energy balance, metabolic stability, fluid regulation, and stress responses, among others. This chapter discusses the adaptive neuroendocrine responses that occur during exercise, pregnancy, starvation, obesity, anorexia nervosa, and chronic renal failure. It further outlines key neuroendocrine diseases and disorders of energy homeostasis, hypothalamic–pituitary–adrenal (HPA) axis dysregulation, and neuroendocrine tumors.

**Keywords**

Neuroendocrine system · Homeostasis · Exercise · Pregnancy · Obesity · Anorexia nervosa · Neuroendocrine tumors · Chronic renal failure

## 12.1 Introduction

The neuroendocrine system is one of the most prominent regulatory systems of the human body, playing a crucial role in maintaining homeostasis. This bidirectional communication between neural networks and the endocrine system is essential for sustaining overall health and well-being.

At the core of this system lies the hypothalamus, a key neural integrator responsible for regulating vital functions such as food intake, thirst, body temperature, and circadian rhythms. It receives and processes signals from various brain regions and

M. Kaur (✉)
Department of Physiology, VMMC and Safdarjung Hospital, New Delhi, India





H. Prabhakar, M. Kaur (eds.), *Brain and Endocrine Crosstalk*, Physiology in Clinical Neurosciences – Brain and Spinal Cord Crosstalks,
https://doi.org/10.1007/978-981-92-0763-3_12

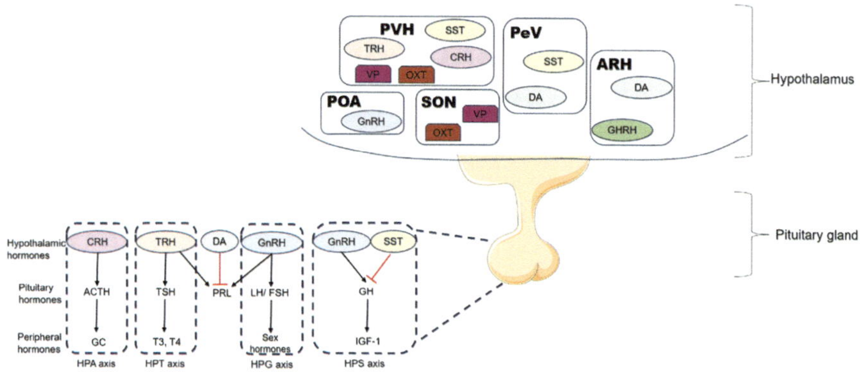


**Fig. 12.1** The neuroendocrine axis with the hypothalamus, pituitary, and peripheral gland along with the hormones involved. *PVH* paraventricular nucleus of the hypothalamus, *POA* preoptic area, *SON* supraoptic nucleus, *PeV* periventricular nucleus, *ARH* arcuate nucleus of the hypothalamus, *TRH* thyrotropin-releasing hormone, *SST* somatostatin, *CRH* corticotropin-releasing hormone, *VP* vasopressin, *OXT* oxytocin, *GnRH* gonadotropin-releasing hormone, *DA* dopamine, *GHRH* growth hormone-releasing hormone, *ACTH* adrenocorticotropic hormone, *GC* glucocorticoids, *TSH* thyroid-stimulating hormone, *T3, T4* thyroid hormones, *PRL* prolactin, *LH* luteinizing hormone, *FSH* follicle-stimulating hormone, *GH* growth hormone, *IGF-1* insulin-like growth factor-1, *HPA* hypothalamic–pituitary–adrenal, *HPT* hypothalamic–pituitary–thyroid, *HPG* hypothalamic–pituitary–gonadal, *HPS* hypothalamic–pituitary–somatotropic

initiates appropriate physiological responses through the endocrine system by producing and releasing neurohormones.

Working closely with the hypothalamus is the pituitary gland, the "master gland," which synthesizes and secretes a wide range of hormones that influence other endocrine organs. These include growth hormone, thyroid-stimulating hormone, adrenocorticotropic hormone, follicle-stimulating hormone, luteinizing hormone, prolactin, and oxytocin, among others.

The neuroendocrine axis extends further to peripheral glands such as the thyroid, adrenal glands, pancreas, and gonads (ovaries and testes). Through these organs, it regulates fundamental physiological processes including metabolism, stress responses, reproduction, growth, and development, among other functions.

Importantly, endocrine hormones provide reciprocal feedback to the hypothalamus and pituitary through complex regulatory loops (Fig. 12.1). This ensures that the system maintains an intricate balance and is responding appropriately to internal and external cues.

This chapter will explore the neuroendocrine adaptations associated with a few of the physiological and clinical conditions.

## 12.2 Physiological Conditions

### 12.2.1 Exercise

Exercise functions as both a stressor and a modifier of stress within the neuroendocrine system. During acute physical activity, the neuroendocrine system faces two primary challenges: the regulation of energy metabolism and the maintenance of body fluids and electrolytes. Exercise induces changes in the circulating levels of many hormones from their baseline values (as shown in Table 12.1) [1]. Most of these hormones serve as mediators of stress to varying degrees.

However, the principal stress-related hormones are those linked to the sympathetic nervous system and the hypothalamic–pituitary–adrenocortical–adrenomedullary (HPA-A) axis—namely norepinephrine, epinephrine, adrenocorticotropic hormone (ACTH), and cortisol.

Despite the acute rise in these hormones during exercise, chronic regular exercise results in an attenuation of the neuroendocrine stress response, reflecting improved physiological resilience and adaptation.

The activation of the HPA axis stimulates the release of corticotropin-releasing hormone (CRH), which further causes the release of ACTH from the anterior pituitary. ACTH acts on the adrenal cortex, augmenting the release of cortisol. Finally, cortisol supports gluconeogenesis and lipolysis, and helps maintain blood pressure during exercise.

The sympathetic–adrenomedullary system releases catecholamines that increase heart rate, cardiac output, blood glucose, and lipolysis during exercise.

Growth hormone (GH) release increases in a pulsatile manner during moderate-to-high-intensity exercise. β-Endorphins rise, contributing to analgesia and perceived well-being.

Arginine vasopressin (AVP) increases due to sweat loss and rising plasma osmolality. Additionally, renin–angiotensin–aldosterone (RAAS) activation enhances sodium and water retention.

As the exercise intensity increases, there is a proportionate increase in the circulating concentrations of stress hormones. This is called the volume effect [2]. However, there lies a critical intensity threshold of approximately 50–60% of

**Table 12.1** Hormones affected substantially by an acute exercise session

| |
|---|
| Adrenocorticotropic hormone |
| Atrial natriuretic peptide |
| Arginine vasopressin |
| β-Endorphin |
| Brain natriuretic peptide |
| Corticotropin-releasing hormone |
| Cortisol |
| Cytokines |
| Dynorphins |
| Enkephalins |
| Epinephrine |
| Growth hormone |
| Norepinephrine |
| Prolactin |
| Renin–angiotensin–aldosterone |
| Testosterone |

maximal oxygen uptake ($VO_2$ max) before these hormones demonstrate a significant elevation in their levels.

If the exercise intensity is held constant but the duration of exercise is increased, it is seen to further augment the hormonal stress response. This progressive rise is likely to be multifactorial, including factors such as hemoconcentration, increased hormone production, and reduced metabolic clearance [3].

After exercise training, an interesting phenomenon of an augmented stress-hormone response is observed during maximal exercise. Two factors may possibly contribute to this effect:

1. A higher absolute workload is required to reach the maximal effort in trained individuals.
2. The development of glandular adaptations enhances the secretory capacity of the endocrine organs [4].

At the same time, chronic exercise training leads to a lower neuroendocrine response to non-exercise stressors. For example, Traustadottir et al. demonstrated that physically active women displayed a markedly lower cortisol response to a standardized psychosocial stressor compared with sedentary women [5]. With training, the following beneficial neuroendocrine adaptations are observed:

1. There is reduced basal and stress-induced cortisol. This reflects the enhanced physiological resilience and improved HPA regulation.
2. They exhibit lower sympathetic activity with enhanced vagal modulations at rest, which improves the cardiovascular recovery.
3. Improvement in anabolic–catabolic balance with enhancement in GH/IGF-1 axis function and insulin sensitivity. Chronic endurance training improves the utilization of lipids over carbohydrates.

However, the adaptability of the neuroendocrine system has limits. Excessive training can drive the stress response into a maladaptive zone, increasing the risk of chronic fatigue and the development of overtraining syndrome.

### 12.2.2 Pregnancy

Pregnancy is a special physiological state where varied neuroendocrine adaptations occur so as to help in sustaining fetal growth, maintaining maternal homeostasis, and preparing the body for parturition and lactation. These adaptations are coordinated primarily by the hypothalamus, which integrates hormonal, metabolic, and behavioral signals and governs downstream endocrine responses through its control of the pituitary and peripheral endocrine organs.

Pregnancy involves a complex interplay between three major components—the mother, the placenta, and the fetus. This triad produces and modulates a wide range

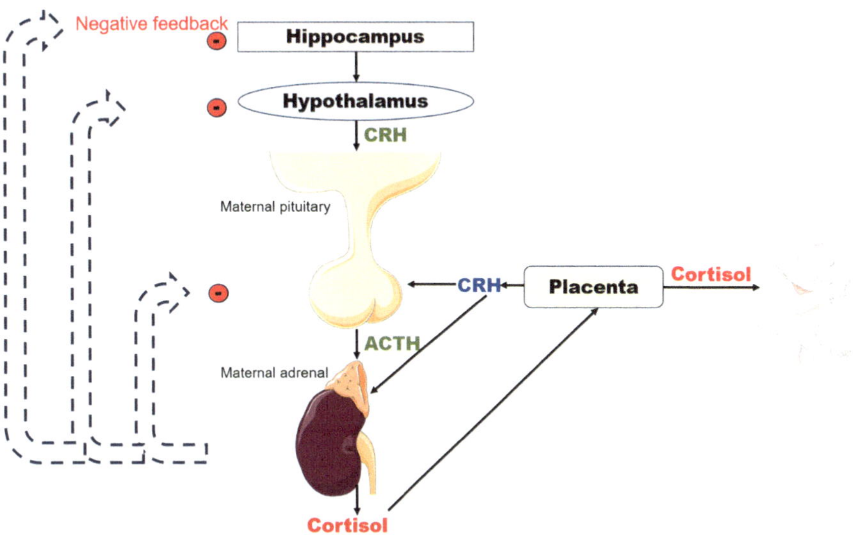


**Fig. 12.2** Neuroendocrine adaptations of HPA axis in pregnancy. *CRH* corticotropin-releasing hormone, *ACTH* adrenocorticotropic hormone

of hormones required for maintaining gestation. The following neuroendocrine axis adaptations have been widely observed in pregnancy.

#### 12.2.2.1 Hypothalamic–Pituitary–Adrenal (HPA) Axis

The HPA axis becomes progressively activated throughout gestation. Maternal cortisol levels rise steadily, driven in part by placental corticotropin-releasing hormone (CRH). Elevated cortisol supports fetal organ maturation, modulates maternal glucose metabolism, and contributes to insulin resistance—a normal adaptation to ensure fetal nutrient supply [6].

However, excessive cortisol reactivity and high maternal stress exposure have been linked to negative outcomes for both mother and fetus, including increased risk of depression, impaired physical health, and alterations in fetal neurodevelopment (Fig. 12.2).

#### 12.2.2.2 Hypothalamic–Pituitary–Thyroid (HPT) Axis

The HPT axis undergoes significant modification in early pregnancy. Rising estrogen stimulates an increase in thyroid-binding globulin, while human chorionic gonadotropin (hCG) transiently activates thyroid hormone production. These changes enhance maternal metabolic rate and thermogenesis, ensuring adequate energy availability.

Importantly, women with hypothyroxinemia in early gestation face increased risk for cognitive decline during pregnancy, even when controlling for depression and sleep problems [7].

#### 12.2.2.3 Hypothalamic–Pituitary–Gonadal (HPG) Axis

The HPG axis drives dramatic increases in estrogen and progesterone, which regulate implantation, maintain uterine quiescence, modulate maternal immunity, and induce metabolic changes including fat deposition and insulin resistance. These adaptations ensure that adequate energy substrates are routed to the fetus.

#### 12.2.2.4 Oxytocin–Vasopressin Systems

Oxytocin and vasopressin pathways undergo critical changes to regulate maternal fluid balance, fetal cardiovascular adaptations, onset of labor, maternal bonding, and postpartum milk ejection [8].

#### 12.2.2.5 Neuroendocrine Regulation of Appetite and Metabolism

Pregnancy is characterized by a shift toward positive energy balance. Hypothalamic circuits involving orexigenic (NPY/AgRP) and anorexigenic (POMC) neurons are modulated by circulating and placental hormones such as:

- Human placental lactogen (hPL)
- Placental growth hormone
- Leptin (with partial leptin resistance)
- Progesterone and estrogen

These adaptations ensure increased maternal appetite, enhanced fat storage, and insulin resistance—physiological mechanisms that guarantee nutrient allocation to the fetus [9].

The profound hormonal fluctuations during pregnancy can disrupt circadian rhythms, leading to insomnia, especially in mid-to-late gestation. Insomnia is strongly associated with depressive symptoms, anxiety, and suicidal ideation [10].

Not only do sex steroid fluctuations influence mood but also cortisol dysregulation contributes to perinatal depressive symptoms. High maternal stress, as noted, adversely impacts both maternal well-being and fetal development.

The magnitude of neuroendocrine changes provides important insight into pregnancy-related clinical disorders, including gestational diabetes mellitus, preeclampsia, thyroid disorders of pregnancy, perinatal depression, and anxiety along with postpartum endocrine dysregulation.

## 12.3 Pathological Conditions

### 12.3.1 Starvation and Anorexia Nervosa

The regulation of appetite and metabolism is governed by a complex and highly integrated neuroendocrine network that coordinates central neural circuits with peripheral hormonal signals to maintain energy balance. At the core of this regulatory system lies the hypothalamus, which integrates nutrient, hormonal, and neural inputs to generate adaptive responses related to feeding behavior, energy expenditure, and metabolic homeostasis. Key hypothalamic nuclei—including the arcuate nucleus (ARH), paraventricular nucleus (PVH), lateral hypothalamic area (LHA), and ventromedial hypothalamus (VMH)—contain specialized neuronal populations whose interactions form the foundation of appetite control (Fig. 12.3).

Two major, functionally opposing neuronal populations in the ARH orchestrate energy intake:

(A) Agouti-related peptide (AgRP)/neuropeptide Y (NPY) neurons, which promote hunger and decrease energy expenditure
(B) Proopiomelanocortin (POMC) neurons, which suppress appetite and enhance energy expenditure

These neurons respond to peripheral metabolic cues including leptin, insulin, ghrelin, thyroid hormones, and glucocorticoids, enabling the hypothalamus to dynamically regulate feeding under various physiological and pathological conditions. Emerging evidence shows that many neuroendocrine cells traditionally considered purely endocrine—such as corticotropin-releasing hormone (CRH), thyrotropinreleasing hormone (TRH), and oxytocin/vasopressin neurons—also exert non-endocrine metabolic influences through glutamatergic or GABAergic neural circuits, adding complexity to classical neuroendocrine models [11].

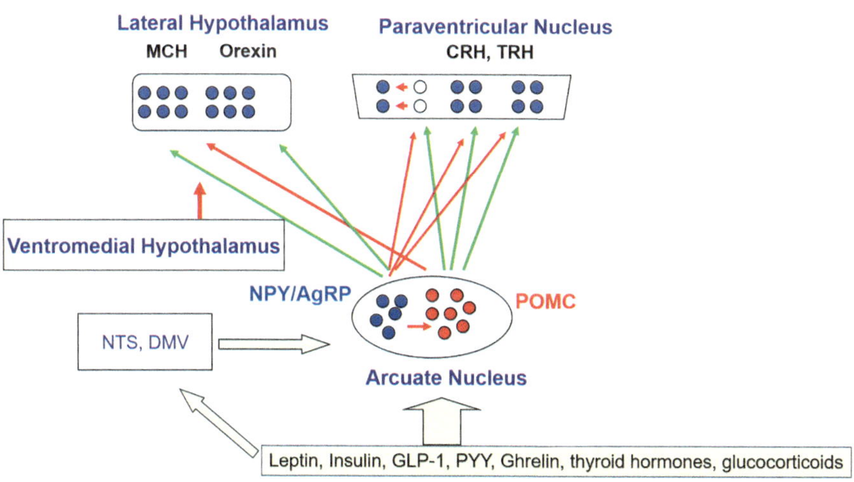


**Fig. 12.3** The neuroendocrinological control of appetite. *MCH* melanin-concentrating hormone, *CRH* corticotropin-releasing hormone, *TRH* thyrotropin-releasing hormone, *NPY* neuropeptide Y, *AgRP* agouti related protein, *POMC* proopiomelanocortin, *NTS* nucleus tractus solitarius, *DMV* dorsal nucleus of vagus, *GLP-1* glucagon-like peptide-1, *PYY* peptide YY

#### 12.3.1.1 Neuroendocrine Responses to Starvation

Starvation triggers a coordinated hormonal and behavioral response aimed at preserving energy for vital organs. The fall in glucose and insulin, together with elevated ghrelin, leads to strong activation of AgRP/NPY neurons, increasing hunger drive. Simultaneously, reduced leptin and insulin levels decrease POMC neuronal activity, removing anorexigenic tone.

Additional adaptations include:

- HPA axis activation → increased cortisol, promoting hepatic gluconeogenesis and lipolysis. Chronic glucocorticoid elevation enhances appetite and fat deposition when food becomes available.
- HPT axis suppression → reduced T3/T4 production and decreased thermogenesis to conserve energy.
- Reduced sympathetic outflow to brown adipose tissue (BAT) → decreased UCP1-mediated heat production.

At the neural level, fasting increases hypothalamic Adenosine Monophosphate-activated Protein Kinase (AMPK) activation, which enhances feeding drive via stimulation of NPY/AgRP circuits and preferential carbohydrate seeking during refeeding [12].

Besides this, HPA and HPT axes exert potent metabolic effects beyond their classical endocrine functions. Glucocorticoids enhance feeding, increase fat mass, and alter lipid metabolism, while central administration of ACTH or CRH tends to reduce food intake and enhance energy expenditure, highlighting distinct central vs. peripheral actions. Similarly, thyroid hormones elevate metabolic rate and modulate feeding behavior through AMPK-dependent mechanisms in the VMH, whereas TRH can exert anorexigenic effects independent of thyroid hormone release. These dual modes of action underscore the complex interplay between neuroendocrine hormones and neural circuits in maintaining energy homeostasis.

#### 12.3.1.2 Neuroendocrine Dysregulation in Anorexia

Anorexia nervosa represents an extreme maladaptation in which neuroendocrine mechanisms designed for short-term starvation remain persistently activated [13, 14]. Chronic caloric deficiency leads to:

- Marked suppression of leptin, maintaining chronic AgRP/NPY activation and reduced POMC activity—yet behavioral eating remains suppressed due to higher-order cognitive circuits overriding hypothalamic homeostasis.
- Elevated CRH in central stress pathways, contributing to hyperactivity and appetite suppression. Experimental CRH administration decreases food intake and increases thermogenesis via sympathetic pathways.
- Hypothalamic amenorrhea due to reduced GnRH pulsatility and suppression of the HPG axis.
- Suppressed thyroid function (low T3) despite normal TSH, reflecting adaptation to conserve energy.

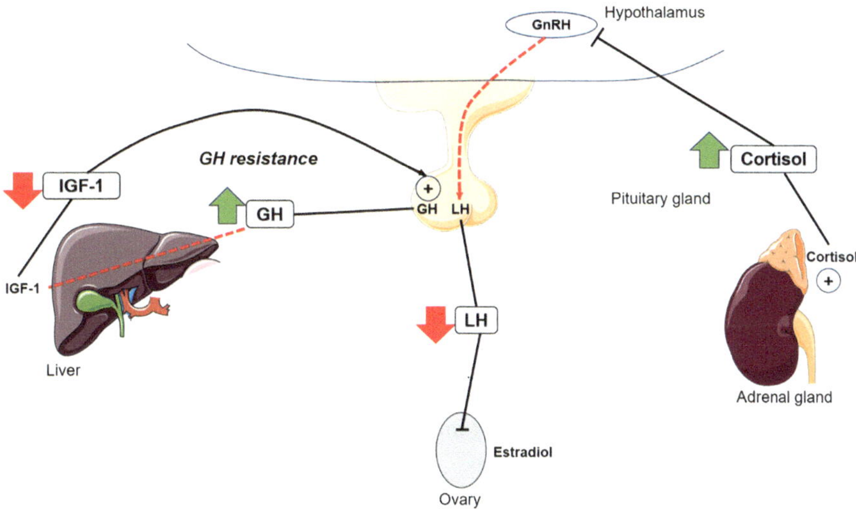


**Fig. 12.4** Neuroendocrine adaptations in anorexia. Chronic undernutrition in this condition causes hypercortisolemia, functional hypothalamic amenorrhea (hypogonadotropic hypogonadism), and growth hormone (GH) resistance. *GnRH* gonadotropin releasing hormone, *LH* luteinizing hormone, *GH* growth hormone, *IGF-1* insulin-like growth factor 1

These dysregulated neuroendocrine pathways sustain reduced appetite, impaired metabolic rate, and altered stress responsiveness characteristic of anorexia (Fig. 12.4).

### 12.3.2 Obesity

Obesity results from chronic positive energy balance, but is sustained by profound neuroendocrine reprogramming within the hypothalamus [15, 16]:

- Leptin resistance, rather than leptin deficiency, is central. High leptin levels fail to inhibit AgRP neurons or stimulate POMC neurons effectively.
- Insulin resistance in hypothalamic neurons further disrupts appetite control.
- Blunted PVH CRH neuronal responsiveness has been shown to predispose to diet-induced obesity by impairing satiety signaling and energy expenditure.
- Hypothalamic inflammation from chronic high-fat feeding alters synaptic organization of metabolic circuits, weakening anorexigenic pathways.
- Elevated glucocorticoids promote hyperphagia and weight gain by modulating ARH neurons and increasing visceral adiposity.
- Peripheral endocrine changes—such as increased insulin and altered adipokine profiles—further reinforce central resistance to anorexigenic signals.

### 12.3.3 Neuroendocrine Diseases

Neuroendocrine diseases are an umbrella term for a spectrum of disorders affecting the complex interactions between the nervous system and the endocrine system. Several conditions are now classified under the category of neuroendocrine diseases, including diabetes insipidus, Kallmann syndrome, rheumatoid arthritis, and many others. We will briefly discuss a few representative examples.

#### 12.3.3.1 Disorders of Energy Homeostasis

- Leptin and leptin receptor deficiencies

Leptin plays an important role in the regulation of body weight by affecting glucose and lipid homeostasis along with appetite and energy expenditure [17, 18]. Thus, defects in leptin or its receptor may lead to hypothalamic resistance to metabolic cues and contribute to diabetes.

Severe insulin resistance, as observed in lipodystrophic mice and humans, can be partly corrected by leptin replacement therapy [19, 20]. These antidiabetic actions are believed to be mediated primarily in the arcuate nucleus of the hypothalamus.

- Obesity due to defective melanocortin signaling

Mutations in the proopiomelanocortin (*POMC*) gene are associated with a rare human syndrome characterized by ACTH insufficiency, red hair pigmentation, and early-onset obesity. This clinical picture arises from a deficiency of circulating ACTH and the absence of melanocortin peptides in both the skin and the brain [21]. These findings provide strong evidence that central melanocortin pathways play a critical role in human energy homeostasis.

Further support came from the discovery of heterozygous frameshift mutations in the melanocortin-4 receptor (*MC4R*) gene, associated with non-syndromic obesity. Affected individuals exhibit increased adiposity, accelerated linear growth, increased lean mass, hyperinsulinemia disproportionate to their degree of obesity, and severe hyperphagia [22, 23].

#### 12.3.3.2 Neuropsychiatric Disorders

Functional alterations in key neural centers—including the hippocampus, prefrontal cortex, and amygdala—can profoundly influence hypothalamic–pituitary–adrenal (HPA) axis function. Dysregulation of this axis has strong associations with several mood and affective disorders, such as major depression and post-traumatic stress disorder (PTSD) [24, 25]. Eating disorders like anorexia nervosa also represent classic conditions with complex neuroendocrine involvement.

#### 12.3.3.3 Neuroendocrine Tumors

Neuroendocrine neoplasms constitute a diverse group of tumors that may secrete bioactive hormones or bioamines, depending on their site of origin, differentiation, and functional status. These tumors can produce distinctive paraneoplastic syndromes, such as carcinoid syndrome, Cushing syndrome, and Zollinger–Ellison syndrome. Common sites of origin include the lung, pancreas, and prostate [26].

### 12.3.4 Chronic Renal Failure

Chronic renal failure causes major disturbances in fluid balance, electrolyte handling, acid–base homeostasis, blood pressure regulation, and metabolism [27]. To compensate, multiple neuroendocrine systems become activated (Table 12.2). These adaptations are initially helpful but later contribute to complications:

(A) Renin–Angiotensin–Aldosterone System (RAAS) Activation

- Reduced renal perfusion + decreased sodium delivery to macula densa → increased renin release.
- ↑ Angiotensin II → vasoconstriction, maintains Glomerular Filtration Rate (GFR) by efferent arteriole constriction.
- ↑ Aldosterone → promotes $Na^+$ and water retention.
- Long-term effect: Hypertension, LV hypertrophy, glomerular hypertension → accelerates nephron loss.

(B) Sympathetic Nervous System (SNS) Overactivity

- Reduced renal blood flow stimulates renal sympathetic nerves.
- ↑ Norepinephrine → systemic vasoconstriction → helps maintain BP.
- Long-term effect: Resistant hypertension, cardiac arrhythmias, impaired baroreflex function.

(C) Antidiuretic Hormone (ADH)/Vasopressin

- Reduced ability to concentrate/dilute urine due to nephron loss.

**Table 12.2** Neuroendocrine adaptations in chronic renal failure

| System | Change | Purpose | Long-term harm |
|---|---|---|---|
| Renin–angiotensin–aldosterone system | ↑ Renin, Ang II, aldosterone | Maintain BP, GFR | Hypertension, fibrosis |
| Sympathetic nervous system | ↑ Tone | Maintain perfusion | Left ventricular hypertrophy, arrhythmias |
| Anti-diuretic hormone | ↑ | Water retention | Fluid overload |
| Natriuretic peptides | ↑ But resistant | Promote natriuresis | No major benefit |
| Parathyroid hormone | ↑ | Correct Ca–P balance | Bone/vascular disease |
| Erythropoietin | ↓ | – | Anemia |
| Growth hormone | ↑ GH, ↓ IGF-1 | Growth | Growth failure |
| Gonadal hormones | ↓ Sex hormones | – | Infertility |
| Prolactin | ↑ | – | Sexual dysfunction |

- Chronic mild hypovolemia, hyperosmolarity → ↑ ADH secretion.
- Promotes water reabsorption in remaining nephrons.
- Long-term effect: Dilutional hyponatremia, increased fluid overload.

(D) Natriuretic Peptides (ANP and BNP)

- Volume expansion and stretch of cardiac atria/ventricles → ↑ ANP and BNP.
- Promotes natriuresis, vasodilation → attempts to counter RAAS/SNS.
- But reduced renal responsiveness due to nephron loss → resistance to natriuretic peptides.

(E) Parathyroid Hormone (PTH)
Part of mineral metabolism disturbance:

- ↓ GFR → phosphate retention → hyperphosphatemia.
- ↓ Active vitamin D (1,25-$(OH)_2$ $D_3$) synthesis.
- → Hypocalcemia → ↑ PTH secretion (secondary hyperparathyroidism).
- Effects: Bone disease, vascular calcification, neuromuscular dysfunction.

(F) Insulin and Glucose Metabolism

- Reduced renal insulin clearance → ↑ plasma insulin levels.
- Peripheral insulin resistance increases.
- Outcome: Glucose intolerance but sometimes less insulin requirement in diabetics.

(G) Erythropoietin (EPO)

- Diseased kidneys → decreased EPO production.
- Leads to normocytic, normochromic anemia → fatigue, cardiac stress.

(H) Growth Hormone (GH)—IGF-1 Axis

- GH levels elevated due to reduced renal clearance.
- But peripheral GH resistance → reduced IGF-1 levels.
- Outcome: Growth retardation in children with CRF.

(I) Hypothalamic–Pituitary–Gonadal Axis

- Uremia disrupts GnRH pulsatility.
- ↓ LH, FSH secretion → hypogonadism, menstrual irregularities, reduced fertility.
- Males → ↓ testosterone, impotence.

(J) Prolactin

- Reduced renal clearance → hyperprolactinemia.
- Contributes to sexual dysfunction, gynecomastia.

(K) Cortisol and Thyroid Hormones

- Cortisol: Normal secretion but reduced clearance → mildly elevated levels.
- Thyroid: "Euthyroid sick syndrome."
  - ↓ T3, normal or low-normal T4.
  - TSH usually normal.

## References


1. Hackney AC. Stress and the neuroendocrine system: the role of exercise as a stressor and modifier of stress. Expert Rev Endocrinol Metab. 2006;1(6):783–92.
2. Viru A. Plasma hormones and physical exercise. Int J Sports Med. 1992;13:201–9.
3. McMurray RG, Hackney AC. Endocrine responses to exercise and training. In: Garrett W, editor. Exercise and sport science. Philadelphia: Lippincott Williams & Wilkins; 2000. p. 135–62.
4. Park E, Chan O, Li Q, et al. Changes in basal hypothalamic–pituitary–adrenal activity during exercise are centrally mediated. Am J Physiol Regul Integr Comp Physiol. 2005;289:R1360–71.
5. Traustadottir T, Bosch PR, Matt KS. The HPA axis response to stress in women: effects of aging and fitness. Psychoneuroendocrinology. 2005;30:392–402.
6. Duthie L, Reynolds RM. Changes in the maternal hypothalamic–pituitary–adrenal axis in pregnancy and postpartum: influences on maternal and fetal outcomes. Neuroendocrinology. 2013;98(2):106–15.
7. Brown EDL, Obeng-Gyasi B, Hall JE, Shekhar S. The thyroid hormone axis and female reproduction. Int J Mol Sci. 2023;24(12):9815.
8. Szczepanska-Sadowska E, Cudnoch-Jedrzejewska A, Wsol A. The role of oxytocin and vasopressin in the pathophysiology of heart failure in pregnancy and in fetal and neonatal life. Am J Physiol Heart Circ Physiol. 2020;318(3):H639–51.
9. Douglas AJ, Johnstone LE, Leng G. Neuroendocrine mechanisms of change in food intake during pregnancy: a potential role for brain oxytocin. Physiol Behav. 2007;91(4):352–65.
10. Trifu S, Vladuti A, Popescu A. The neuroendocrinological aspects of pregnancy and postpartum depression. Acta Endocrinol (Buchar). 2019;15(3):410–5.
11. Yoo ES, Yu J, Sohn JW. Neuroendocrine control of appetite and metabolism. Exp Mol Med. 2021;53:505–16.
12. Amorim T, Khiyami A, Latif T, Fazeli PK. Neuroendocrine adaptations to starvation. Psychoneuroendocrinology. 2023;157:106365.
13. Schorr M, Miller KK. The endocrine manifestations of anorexia nervosa: mechanisms and management. Nat Rev Endocrinol. 2017;13(3):174–86.
14. Misra M, Klibanski A. Neuroendocrine consequences of anorexia nervosa in adolescents. Endocr Dev. 2010;17:197–214.
15. Chamarthi VS, Daley SF. Obesity as a chronic disease: epidemiology and pathophysiologic insights. In: StatPearls [Internet]. Treasure Island: StatPearls Publishing; 2025.
16. Makki K, Froguel P, Wolowczuk I. Adipose tissue in obesity-related inflammation and insulin resistance: cells, cytokines, and chemokines. ISRN Inflamm. 2013;2013:139239.
17. Elmquist JK, Marcus JN. Rethinking the central causes of diabetes. Nat Med. 2003;9(6):645–7.
18. Elmquist JK, Coppari R, Balthasar N, Ichinose M, Lowell BB. Identifying hypothalamic pathways controlling food intake, body weight, and glucose homeostasis. J Comp Neurol. 2005;493(1):63–71.
19. Shimomura I, Hammer RE, Ikemoto S, Brown MS, Goldstein JL. Leptin reverses insulin resistance and diabetes mellitus in mice with congenital lipodystrophy. Nature. 1999;401(6748):73–6.
20. Ebihara K, Ogawa Y, Masuzaki H, et al. Transgenic overexpression of leptin rescues insulin resistance and diabetes in a mouse model of lipoatrophic diabetes. Diabetes. 2001;50(6):1440–8.

21. Krude H, Biebermann H, Luck W, Horn R, Brabant G, Grüters A. Severe early-onset obesity, adrenal insufficiency and red hair pigmentation caused by POMC mutations in humans. Nat Genet. 1998;19(2):155–7.
22. Farooqi IS, Keogh JM, Yeo GSH, Lank EJ, Cheetham T, O'Rahilly S. Clinical spectrum of obesity and mutations in the melanocortin 4 receptor gene. N Engl J Med. 2003;348(12):1085–95.
23. Branson R, Potoczna N, Kral JG, Lentes KU, Hoehe MR, Horber FF. Binge eating as a major phenotype of melanocortin 4 receptor gene mutations. N Engl J Med. 2003;348(12):1096–103.
24. Herman JP, Mueller NK. Role of the ventral subiculum in stress integration. Behav Brain Res. 2006;174(2):215–24.
25. McKlveen JM, Myers B, Herman JP. The medial prefrontal cortex: coordinator of autonomic, neuroendocrine and behavioural responses to stress. J Neuroendocrinol. 2015;27(6):446–56.
26. Oronsky B, Ma PC, Morgensztern D, Carter CA. Nothing but NET: a review of neuroendocrine tumors and carcinomas. Neoplasia. 2017;19(12):991–1002.
27. Feneberg R, Schaefer F, Veldhuis JD. Neuroendocrine adaptations in renal disease. Pediatr Nephrol. 2003;18(6):492–7.

# Part III

# Brain and Endocrine Crosstalk

# Brain and Endocrine Crosstalk: Clinical Implication for Neurocritical Care

13

Tulskii Ivan, Kulikov Alexander, and Savin Ivan

**Abstract**

Functional interaction between the nervous and endocrine systems plays a crucial role in sodium and water balance regulation, steroid production, glucose metabolism, and thyroid function. The crosstalk between the brain and the endocrine system is particularly evident in various forms of brain injury, including traumatic brain injury, hemorrhage, or tumors. This chapter describes different forms of brain–endocrine crosstalk, with special focus on the clinical implications of this interaction in perioperative medicine and neurocritical care.

**Keywords**

Neurocritical care · Hypothalamic–pituitary–adrenal axis · Brain tumors · Adrenal insufficiency · Diabetes insipidus · Syndrome of inappropriate antidiuretic hormone secretion · Cerebral salt-wasting syndrome · Paroxysmal sympathetic hyperactivity

## 13.1 Introduction

The nervous and endocrine systems are the key elements of the body's internal balance and coordination and respond to external stimuli. Functional interaction between these systems makes brain–endocrine crosstalk inevitable. The most straightforward path of brain impact on the endocrine system is the hypothalamic–pituitary–adrenal (HPA) axis. This structure plays a crucial role in sodium and water

T. Ivan · K. Alexander (✉) · S. Ivan
Burdenko National Medical Research Center of Neurosurgery, Moscow, Russia
e-mail: akulikov@nsi.ru





H. Prabhakar, M. Kaur (eds.), *Brain and Endocrine Crosstalk*, Physiology in Clinical Neurosciences – Brain and Spinal Cord Crosstalks,
https://doi.org/10.1007/978-981-92-0763-3_13

balance regulation, steroid production, glucose metabolism, and thyroid function. Various brain pathologies, including traumatic brain injury, hemorrhage, or tumors, result in endocrine disorders, and, conversely, endocrine disorders can influence normal brain function [1–4].

This chapter describes different forms of brain–endocrine crosstalk, with special focus on the clinical implications of this interaction in perioperative medicine and neurocritical care.

## 13.2 Brain Injury and Endocrine Disorders

The crosstalk between the brain and the endocrine system is particularly evident in various forms of brain injury. In general, the severity of endocrine disorders depends on the nature and extent of involvement of the principal integrative hub of the nervous and endocrine systems—the hypothalamic–pituitary axis or, in a broader context, the diencephalic region. Dysfunction of this system may be caused by direct anatomical damage, secondary ischemic injury, extrinsic compression, or tumor in situ. Depending on the damaging factor, it can lead to suppression of cellular secretory function or, conversely, a pathological increase of secretory activity (Fig. 13.1).

Traumatic brain injury (TBI) can cause direct structural damage to the hypothalamic–pituitary complex, or functional disruption between cortical

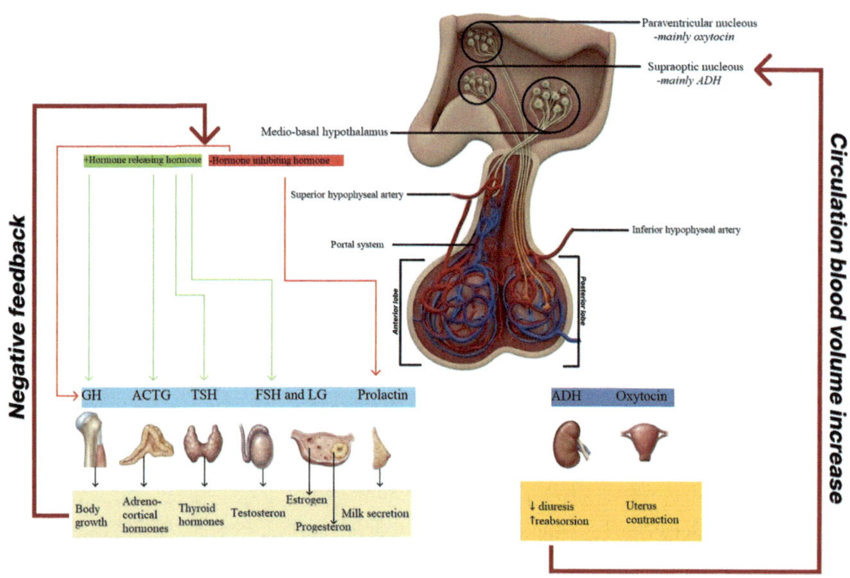


**Fig. 13.1** Functional structure of hypothalamic–pituitary–adrenal axis. *ADH* antidiuretic hormone, *GH* growth hormone, *TSH* thyroid-stimulating hormone, *FSH* follicle-stimulating hormone, *LG* luteinizing hormone, *ACTG* adrenocorticotropic hormone

structures, the brainstem, and the HPA. Moreover, skull fracture, edema, and acute hemorrhage can lead to intracranial hypertension and consequent hypothalamic–pituitary injury. Damage to the hypothalamus and pituitary can also result from TBI-induced hypoxia, hypotension, and secondary ischemia. This type of injury particularly affects the long hypophyseal vessels and the portal capillaries in the pituitary stalk, which lead to anterior lobe infarction. The posterior lobe is less susceptible to injury through this mechanism, because the blood supply to the posterior pituitary is derived from the short hypophyseal vessels [5–17].

The mechanism of subarachnoid hemorrhage (SAH)-induced endocrine disorders relates to the proximity of the circle of Willis to the hypothalamic–pituitary complex. Blood spreading over the skull base in the initial phase of SAH can provoke irritation of diencephalic structures. Direct compression of the pituitary by the aneurysm, vasospasm-induced secondary ischemic injury, increased intracranial pressure, or a surgical procedure can also dramatically alter pituitary functions after SAH [18–29].

Tumors of the hypothalamic–pituitary axis can induce various neuroendocrine disorders. Such dysfunctions can be caused by the mass effect or by direct hormonal activity of tumor cells. The most common clinical signs of HPA-associated tumors are presented in Table 13.1 [29–45].

In clinical practice, neurocritical care specialists focus on timely revealing of typical syndromes associated with acute brain injury or neurosurgical intervention for tumor removal. Among such syndromes, in the context of brain–endocrine crosstalk, are hypopituitarism and secondary adrenal insufficiency, specific forms of water–electrolyte imbalance (diabetes insipidus (DI), syndrome of inappropriate antidiuretic hormone (ADH) secretion (SIADH), or cerebral salt-wasting syndrome (CSWS)), and paroxysmal sympathetic hyperactivity.

**Table 13.1** Clinical signs of HPA-associated tumors

| Tumor | Clinical presentation |
|---|---|
| Craniopharyngioma [46–53] | Growth hormone deficiency is the most common sign. Panhypopituitarism or diabetes insipidus appears less often. Clinically, patient presents with headache, visual field defects, dioplopia, and short stature |
| Hypothalamic/optic chiasm glioma [54–57] | The most common disorder are hypopituitarism, precocious puberty, and diencephalic syndrome (a rare cause of failure to thrive in infancy). Hypothalamic or chiasmatic astrocytomas associated with diencephalic syndrome are often larger in size, more aggressive, and may seed throughout the cerebrospinal fluid pathway |
| Hypothalamic hamartoma [58–62] | Clinically, the presenting symptoms include precocious puberty, gelastic (laughing) seizures, and developmental delay |

(continued)

**Table 13.1** (continued)

| Tumor | Clinical presentation |
|---|---|
| Pituitary adenoma [62–110]<br>1. Corticotropinoma<br>2. Prolactinoma<br>3. Somatotropinoma<br>4. Gonadotropinoma<br>5. Thyrotropinoma | Pituitary adenomas may be:<br>• Functional (hormonally active)<br>• Nonfunctional (without measurable hormonal activity)<br>Among hormonally active tumors, adrenocorticotropic hormone (ACTH)-releasing adenomas are most common in the first decade of life, while prolactinomas and growth hormone (GH)-releasing adenomas become more common in the teenage years<br>1. ACTH-releasing adenomas or childhood corticotropinomas associated with Cushing's disease. The most common clinical presentation of Cushing's disease is significant weight gain and severe failure to gain height. Other common symptoms include headache, hypertension, glucose intolerance, delayed puberty, amenorrhea, virilization, and hirsutism<br>2. The symptoms associated with prolactinoma are broadly divided into those that are caused by increased prolactin levels and others that are caused by mass effect. Those that are caused by increased prolactin levels are amenorrhea/galactorrhea in females, hypogonadism, gynecomastia and erectile dysfunction in males, and loss of axillary/pubic hair, while those that are caused by mass effect are bitemporal hemianopsia (due to pressure on optic chiasma), vertigo, nausea, and vomiting. Pituitary apoplexy is characterized by clinical findings of sudden onset headache usually associated with visual disturbance<br>3. Clinical presentation in children and adolescents depends on whether the epiphyseal plate is open or fused. Prior to epiphyseal fusion, overproduction of GH causes giganitism in children, while postepiphyseal fusion and overproduction of GH cause acromegaly in adults. Headache and visual disturbances are not infrequent with somatotropinomas |
| Germinoma [111–116] | Suprasellar germinomas have diabetes insipidus (DI) as one of the presenting symptoms, reflecting involvement of hypothalamus and pituitary stalk |
| Leukemia and lymphoma | Pituitary stalk involvement and thickening have been reported with leukemia (chronic myelogenous leukemia and acute myelogenous leukemia) and lymphoma. Clinically, these patients have DI |
| Rathke's cleft cyst [117–129] | The most common neuroendocrine presentation in Rathke's cyst is hypopituitarism and delayed puberty |

## 13.3 Adrenal Insufficiency

Adrenal insufficiency is an endocrine disorder caused by decreased secretion of glucocorticoid and mineralocorticoid hormones by the adrenal cortex as a result of impaired function or direct injury, including surgical manipulations, of the hypothalamic–pituitary–adrenal axis [130–138]. In patients with neurosurgical pathology, secondary (pituitary injury) or tertiary (hypothalamic injury) adrenal insufficiencies are observed [139–142]. Secondary adrenal insufficiency develops both as a consequence of reduced ACTH production and as a damage to the pituitary stalk. Secondary and tertiary adrenal insufficiencies, typically, develop in combination with deficiencies of the following tropic hormones:

- Luteinizing hormone (LH)
- Thyroid-stimulating hormone (TSH)
- Growth hormone (GH)

Clinical manifestations of adrenal insufficiency in the postoperative period after surgical manipulations in the diencephalic region include:

- Arterial hypotension refractory to fluid loading and sympathomimetic agents
- Cortisol level $\leq$ 410 nmol/L ($\leq$250 nmol/L—critical level)
- Hypoglycemia, hyponatremia, hyperkalemia, and eosinophilia
- Memory impairment, depression, and somnolence
- Systemic inflammatory response without signs of infection
- Multiple organ dysfunction

Glucocorticoid therapy is primarily based on clinical presentation and laboratory data on blood cortisol concentration. Hydrocortisone/cortisone is the optimal agent for replacement. In the postoperative setting, a stress dose of glucocorticoids is administered, corresponding to 150–300 mg of hydrocortisone per day. The drug is administered parenterally every 6 h. Starting on postoperative days 2–3, in clinically stable patients, the total daily hydrocortisone dose is reduced by 10–20 mg per day, with complete discontinuation over 7–10 days.

In patients with neurosurgical pathology, secondary hypothyroidism may be an additional manifestation of hypopituitarism. Clinical signs of hypothyroidism include hypothermia, bradycardia, decreased myocardial contractility, intestinal paresis, and peripheral edema. Laboratory markers of hypothyroidism are reduced plasma levels of free thyroxine and triiodothyronine. Such patients need L-thyroxine at a dose of 1–3 mcg/kg/day for correction.

## 13.4 Diabetes Insipidus

Diabetes insipidus (DI) occurs following damage to hypothalamic neurons due to TBI or surgical removal of tumors located in diencephalic region. It is a result of depression of vasopressin/antidiuretic hormone (arginine vasopressin (AVP)/ADH) secretion, resulting in polyuria (often 250–800 mL/h or 3–20 L/day) and hypernatremia. DI is particularly prognostically ominous, associated with more severe trauma, lower GCS scores, and mortality rates of 57–90%, with the highest mortality (86–90%) in early-onset DI presenting within 3 days of injury. The condition frequently persists only transiently (days to weeks), though a minority of survivors develop permanent central DI requiring long-term desmopressin replacement.

A distinctive feature of pituitary stalk injury is the triphasic response, consisting of three sequential phases. Phase 1 involves ADH deficiency manifesting as polyuria and hypernatremia. Phase 2 follows within days to weeks with robust preformed ADH release, producing SIADH, presenting with hyponatremia and oliguria. Phase 3 concludes with ADH depletion and return to a permanent ADH deficiency if pituitary damage is severe. This triphasic response results from transient pituitary shock, followed by the release of preformed hormone stores and ending with depletion due to neuronal damage.

In clinical practice, the following main diagnostic criteria of DI are used:

- Urine osmolality <200 mOsm/L (typically 50–150), specific gravity <1.005. Failure of urine osmolality to rise above 300 mOsm/L under dehydration conditions
- Polyuria—diuresis rate exceeding 250 mL/h (in children >3 mL/kg/h)
- Plasma sodium elevation in the setting of polyuria
- Thirst with preserved drinking motivation

DI therapy in the early postoperative period includes:

- Hourly monitoring of fluid input volume and urine output
- Plasma Na level and plasma osmolality control every 6 h
- Synthetic vasopressin analogs: Intranasal and oral (sublingual, enteral) forms available, dose titration performed individually
- Water deficit correction
  - Enteral administration—optimal method (orally with preserved drinking motivation; water via nasogastric tube also possible).
  - Intravenous infusion if enteral route unavailable or in hemodynamic instability due to hypovolemia. Crystalloid solutions used for replacement. With high serum sodium, 5% glucose/0.9% NaCl solutions (1:1) may be employed. Caution required with hypoosmolar solutions; switch to isoosmolar solutions upon achieving normal serum sodium concentration.

## 13.5 Syndrome of Inappropriate Antidiuretic Hormone Secretion and Cerebral Salt-Wasting Syndrome

Syndrome of inappropriate ADH secretion (SIADH) develops as a result of excessive entry of vasopressin/ADH to bloodstream [140, 142–144]. It can accompany the acute phase of SAH, when such type of water–electrolyte imbalance is more common than DI and various other intracranial lesions with pituitary damage.

SIADH is associated with decreased diuresis rate and hyponatremia. The main diagnostic criteria for SIADH are:

- Hyponatremia Na <135 mmol/L
- Low blood plasma osmolality < 280 mOsm/L
- Elevated sodium concentration in urine over 180 mmol/L
- Absence of clinical manifestations of hypovolemia
- Possible hyperhydration
- Normal kidney function

- Absence of adrenal insufficiency (absence of arterial hypotension and hyperkalemia)
- Absence of hypothyroidism

Neurological manifestations of SIADH include impaired consciousness and seizures. If plasma sodium decreases gradually and is moderately pronounced ($Na \geq 125$ mmol/L), clinical manifestations may be minimal, with paradoxically strong thirst.

The crucial role in SIADH management is played by differential diagnosis with cerebral salt-wasting syndrome (CSWS). The last one is associated with excessive secretion of natriuretic peptides and leads to hypovolemia (Table 13.2).

Main principles of SIADH correction include:

- Prevent hypernatremia during correction; monitor plasma sodium every 1–3 h and adjust therapy based on results.
- Discontinue therapy if plasma Na rises ≥126 mmol/L over 12 h.
- Discontinue therapy if plasma Na change ≥10 mmol/L over 24 h.
- Do not exceed correction rate ≈1 mmol/L/h.
- Slowly infuse 3% (513 mmol/L) or 5% (856 mmol/L) NaCl solution per above principles (starting rate 25–50 mL/h of 3% NaCl or 1–4 mL/kg/h).
- Concurrently, furosemide (Lasix) may be used to prevent hyperhydration and pulmonary edema.
- Potassium deficit must be corrected.
- Correct concomitant anemia if present.
- Hyponatremia correction must be extremely slow in the presence of hypokalemia, not exceeding 8 mmol/L per day.

CSWS therapy includes [139–145]:

- Strict fluid balance monitoring every 3–6 h
- Replacement of fluid with 0.9% NaCl
- Use of 3% NaCl at 1–3 mL/kg for hyponatremia correction when Na <126 mmol/L
- Fludrocortisone 0.1–0.3 mg/day (up to 0.6–0.8 mg/day) to reduce natriuresis

**Table 13.2** Differential diagnosis between SIADH and CSWS

| Parameters | CSWS | SIADH |
|---|---|---|
| Total blood volume | ↓ Hypovolemia | Normovolemia |
| Na balance | Negative | Negative |
| Dehydratation symptoms | Yes | No |
| Body weight | ↓ | ↑ or unchanged |
| Central venous pressure | ↓ (< 6 $mmH_2O$) | ↑ or in references |
| HCT | ↑ | ↓ or in references |
| Plasma osmolarity | ↓ | ↓ |
| [Na] Urine | ↑↑ | ↑ |
| [K] Plasma | ↑ | ↓ |

It is extremely important that too-slow correction of hyponatremia increases the risk of somatic complications and mortality, while excessively rapid correction of chronic hyponatremia may lead to central pontine and extrapontine myelinolysis (CPM). This syndrome implies osmotic demyelination with injury to the white matter of the pons, as well as other areas of cerebral white matter. Symptoms of CPM are mental disturbances, tetraparesis, and peripheral and central cranial nerve palsies, including pseudobulbar palsy.

## 13.6 Paroxysmal Sympathetic Hyperactivity

One of the most striking manifestations of brain–endocrine crosstalk following acute brain injury is the catecholamine surge, also termed sympathetic storm, dysautonomia, or paroxysmal sympathetic hyperactivity (PSH) [145–151]. This phenomenon involves massive release of catecholamines (epinephrine, norepinephrine, and dopamine) from both central and peripheral sources, resulting from disruption of normal inhibitory control mechanisms in the brainstem and diencephalon.

The magnitude of catecholamine elevation is directly proportional to brain injury severity. Patients with severe TBI (Glasgow Coma Scale [GCS] 3–4) demonstrate catecholamine levels approximately five to eight times higher than controls, while patients with better GCS scores (11–12) show only modest elevation. This neuroendocrine marker provides a quantifiable reflection of brain injury extent and correlates reliably with neurological recovery.

The peripheral manifestations of catecholamine storm include profound tachycardia, hypertension, tachypnea, fever, diaphoresis, and mydriasis. Excessive sympathetic activity initiates complex disorders: elevated catecholamines cause peripheral vasoconstriction producing arterial hypertension and increased intracranial pressure (ICP), increase myocardial oxygen demand, induce direct myocardial injury with potential Takotsubo cardiomyopathy, and trigger cytokine release disturbances causing systemic organ damage.

Clinical trials examining beta-blockers, alpha-2-agonists, and gabapentin for catecholamine attenuation have demonstrated promising results [152–157] with improved Glasgow Coma Scale scores and reduced mortality trends in the treatment group. However, universally accepted effective treatment protocols are currently lacking.

## 13.7 Conclusion

Brain–endocrine crosstalk assumes critical clinical significance in neurocritical care patients, where acute brain injuries and HPA-associated tumors create profound neuroendocrine derangements that directly impact patient outcomes, organ dysfunction, and mortality. Disruption of brain–endocrine interaction is a critical driver of secondary morbidity in neurocritical care, manifesting as central adrenal insufficiency, hypothyroidism, catecholamine storm, and complex water–electrolyte imbalances like DI, SIADH, and CSWS. Effective management relies on the early differentiation of these pathologies to prevent iatrogenic harm such as cerebral edema or osmotic demyelination. Ultimately, stabilizing the neuroendocrine axis through precise hormone replacement and fluid management is essential for maintaining hemodynamic stability and optimizing the conditions for neurological recovery.

## References


1. Emelifeonwu JA, Flower H, Loan JJ, McGivern K, Andrews PJD. Prevalence of anterior pituitary dysfunction twelve months or more following traumatic brain injury in adults: a systematic review and meta-analysis. J Neurotrauma. 2020;37(2):217–26. https://doi.org/10.1089/neu.2018.6349.
2. Szarka N, Szellar D, Kiss S, et al. Effect of growth hormone on neuropsychological outcomes and quality of life of patients with traumatic brain injury: a systematic review. J Neurotrauma. 2021;38(11):1467–83. https://doi.org/10.1089/neu.2020.7265.
3. Aljboor GS, Tulemat A, Al-Saedi AR, Radoi MP, Toader C, Papacocea TM. Acute and chronic hypopituitarism following traumatic brain injury: a systematic review and meta-analysis. Neurosurg Rev. 2024;47(1):841. Published 2024 Nov 11. https://doi.org/10.1007/s10143-024-03088-3.
4. Hannon MJ, Sherlock M, Thompson CJ. Pituitary dysfunction following traumatic brain injury or subarachnoid haemorrhage—in "Endocrine Management in the Intensive Care Unit". Best Pract Res Clin Endocrinol Metab. 2011;25(5):783–98. https://doi.org/10.1016/j.beem.2011.06.001.
5. Kelly DF, Gonzalo ITG, Cohan P, Berman N, Swerdloff RS, Wang C. Hypopituitarism following traumatic brain injury and aneurysmal subarachnoid hemorrhage: a preliminary report. J Neurosurg. Published online 2000. https://doi.org/10.3171/JNS.2000.93.5.0743.
6. Lieberman S, Oberoi AL, Gilkison CR, Masel BE, Urban RJ. Prevalence of neuroendocrine dysfunction in patients recovering from traumatic brain injury. J Clin Endocrinol Metab. Published online 2001. https://doi.org/10.1210/JCEM.86.6.7592.
7. Agha A, Thornton E, O'Kelly P, Tormey W, Phillips J, Thompson CJ. Posterior pituitary dysfunction after traumatic brain injury. J Clin Endocrinol Metab. Published online 2004. https://doi.org/10.1210/JC.2004-1058.
8. Popović V, Pekić S, Pavlović D, et al. Hypopituitarism as a consequence of traumatic brain injury (TBI) and its possible relation with cognitive disabilities and mental distress. J Endocrinol Invest. Published online 2004. https://doi.org/10.1007/BF03345308.
9. Agha A, Rogers B, Sherlock M, et al. Anterior pituitary dysfunction in survivors of traumatic brain injury. J Clin Endocrinol Metab. Published online 2004. https://doi.org/10.1210/JC.2004-0511.
10. Bondanelli M, Marinis L de, Ambrosio MR, et al. Occurrence of pituitary dysfunction following traumatic brain injury. J Neurotrauma. Published online 2004. https://doi.org/10.1089/089771504126971 3.
11. Aimaretti G, Ambrosio MR, Somma C di, et al. Traumatic brain injury and subarachnoid haemorrhage are conditions at high risk for hypopituitarism: screening study at 3 months after the brain injury. Clin Endocrinol (Oxf). Published online 2004. https://doi.org/10.1111/J.1365-2265.2004.02094.X.
12. Agha A, Phillips J, O'Kelly P, Tormey WP, Thompson CJT. The natural history of post-traumatic hypopituitarism: implications for assessment and treatment. Am J Med. Published online 2005. https://doi.org/10.1016/J.AMJMED.2005.02.042.
13. Leal-Cerro A, Flores JMG, Rincon M, et al. Prevalence of hypopituitarism and growth hormone deficiency in adults long-term after severe traumatic brain injury. Clin Endocrinol (Oxf). Published online 2005. https://doi.org/10.1111/J.1365-2265.2005.02250.X.

14. Aimaretti G, Ambrosio MR, Somma C di, et al. Residual pituitary function after brain injury-induced hypopituitarism: a prospective 12-month study. J Clin Endocrinol Metab. Published online 2005. https://doi.org/10.1210/JC.2005-0504.
15. Tanrıverdi F, Senyurek H, Ünlühızarcı K, Selçuklu A, Casanueva FF, Keleştimur F. High risk of hypopituitarism after traumatic brain injury: a prospective investigation of anterior pituitary function in the acute phase and 12 months after trauma. J Clin Endocrinol Metab. Published online 2006. https://doi.org/10.1210/JC.2005-2476.
16. Schneider HJ, Kreitschmann-Andermahr I, Ghigo E, Stalla GK, Agha A. Hypothalamopituitary dysfunction following traumatic brain injury and aneurysmal subarachnoid hemorrhage: a systematic review. JAMA. Published online 2007. https://doi.org/10.1001/JAMA.298.12.1429.
17. Tanrıverdi F, Schneider HJ, Aimaretti G, Masel BE, Casanueva FF, Keleştimur F. Pituitary dysfunction after traumatic brain injury: a clinical and pathophysiological approach. Endocr Rev. Published online 2015. https://doi.org/10.1210/ER.2014-1065.
18. Karamouzis I, Pagano L, Prodam F, et al. Clinical and diagnostic approach to patients with hypopituitarism due to traumatic brain injury (TBI), subarachnoid hemorrhage (SAH), and ischemic stroke (IS). Endocrine. 2016;52(3):441–50. https://doi.org/10.1007/s12020-015-0796-2.
19. Karaca Z, Hacioglu A, Kelestimur F. Neuroendocrine changes after aneurysmal subarachnoid haemorrhage. Pituitary. 2019;22(3):305–21. https://doi.org/10.1007/s11102-018-00932-w.
20. Roe T, Welbourne J, Nikitas N. Endocrine dysregulation in aneurysmal subarachnoid haemorrhage. Br J Neurosurg. 2022;36(3):358–67. https://doi.org/10.1080/02688697.2022.2039378
.
21. Brandt L, Säveland H, Valdemarsson S, Sjöholm H, Reinstrup P. Fatigue after aneurysmal subarachnoid hemorrhage evaluated by pituitary function and 3D-CBF. Acta Neurol Scand. Published online 2004. https://doi.org/10.1046/J.0001-6314.2003.00189.X.
22. Dimopoulou I, Kouyialis AT, Tzanella M, et al. High incidence of neuroendocrine dysfunction in long-term survivors of aneurysmal subarachnoid hemorrhage. Stroke. Published online 2004. https://doi.org/10.1161/01.STR.0000147716.45571.45.
23. Kreitschmann-Andermahr I, Hoff C, Saller B, et al. Prevalence of pituitary deficiency in patients after aneurysmal subarachnoid hemorrhage. J Clin Endocrinol Metab. Published online 2004. https://doi.org/10.1210/JC.2004-0146.
24. Kreitschmann-Andermahr I. Subarachnoid hemorrhage as a cause of hypopituitarism. Pituitary. Published online 2005. https://doi.org/10.1007/S11102-006-.
25. Klose M, Brennum J, Poulsgaard L, Kosteljanetz M, Wagner A, Feldt-Rasmussen U. Hypopituitarism is uncommon after aneurysmal subarachnoid haemorrhage. Clin Endocrinol (Oxf). Published online 2010. https://doi.org/10.1111/J.1365-2265.2010.03791.X.
26. Lanterna LA, Spreafico V, Gritti P, et al. Hypocortisolism in noncomatose patients during the acute phase of subarachnoid hemorrhage. J Stroke Cerebrovasc Dis. Published online 2013. https://doi.org/10.1016/J.JSTROKECEREBROVASDIS.2012.11.002.
27. Gardner CJ, Javadpour M, Stoneley C, et al. Low prevalence of hypopituitarism after subarachnoid haemorrhage using confirmatory testing and with BMI-specific GH cut-off levels. Eur J Endocrinol. Published online 2013. https://doi.org/10.1530/EJE-12-0849.
28. Krewer C, Schneider M, Schneider HJ, et al. neuroendocrine disturbances one to five or more years after traumatic brain injury and aneurysmal subarachnoid hemorrhage: data from the German database on hypopituitarism. J Neurotrauma. Published online 2016. https://doi.org/10.1089/NEU.2015.4109.
29. Chaudhary V, Bano S. Imaging of pediatric pituitary endocrinopathies. Indian J Endocrinol Metab. 2012;16(5):682–91. https://doi.org/10.4103/2230-8210.100635.
30. Saeger W, Lüdecke DK, Buchfelder M, Fahlbusch R, Quabbe HJ, Petersenn S. Pathohistological classification of pituitary tumors: 10 years of experience with the German Pituitary Tumor Registry. Eur J Endocrinol. Published online 2007. https://doi.org/10.1530/EJE.1.02326.

31. Trouillas J, Roy P, Stürm N, et al. A new prognostic clinicopathological classification of pituitary adenomas: a multicentric case–control study of 410 patients with 8 years post-operative follow-up. Acta Neuropathol. Published online 2013. https://doi.org/10.1007/S00401-013-1084-Y.
32. Мелмед Ш. Pituitary-tumor endocrinopathies. N Engl J Med. Published online 2020. https://doi.org/10.1056/NEJMRA1810772.
33. Daly A, Beckers A. The epidemiology of pituitary adenomas. Endocrinol Metab Clin North Am (Print). Published online 2020. https://doi.org/10.1016/J.ECL.2020.04.002.
34. Мелмед Ш, Kaiser UB, Lopes MBS, et al. Clinical biology of the pituitary adenoma. Endocr Rev. Published online 2022. https://doi.org/10.1210/ENDREV/BNAC010.
35. Molitch ME. Diagnosis and treatment of pituitary adenomas: a review. J Am Med Assoc (JAMA). Published online 2017. https://doi.org/10.1001/JAMA.2016.19699.
36. Petersenn S, Fleseriu M, Casanueva FF, et al. Diagnosis and management of prolactin-secreting pituitary adenomas: a Pituitary Society international Consensus Statement. Nat Rev Endocrinol. Published online 2023. https://doi.org/10.1038/S41574-023-00886-5.
37. Tritos NA, Miller KK. Diagnosis and management of pituitary adenomas: a review. J Am Med Assoc (JAMA). Published online 2023. https://doi.org/10.1001/JAMA.2023.5444.
38. Chatzellis E, Alexandraki KI, Androulakis II, Kaltsas G. Aggressive pituitary tumors. Neuroendocrinology. Published online 2015. https://doi.org/10.1159/000371806.
39. Trouillas J, Jaffrain-Rea M, Vasiljevic A, Raverot G, Roncaroli F, Villa C. How to classify pituitary neuroendocrine tumors (PitNET)s in 2020. Cancers (Basel). Published online 2020. https://doi.org/10.3390/CANCERS12020514.
40. Nosé V, Ezzat S, Horváth É, et al. Protocol for the examination of specimens from patients with primary pituitary tumors. Arch Pathol Lab Med. Published online 2011. https://doi.org/10.5858/2010-0470-SAR1.1.
41. Ezzat S, Sylvia L, Couldwell WT, et al. The prevalence of pituitary adenomas. Cancer. Published online 2004. https://doi.org/10.1002/CNCR.20412.
42. Sylvia L, Casar-Borota O, Chanson P, et al. From pituitary adenoma to pituitary neuroendocrine tumor (PitNET): an International Pituitary Pathology Club proposal. Endocr Relat Cancer. Published online 2017. https://doi.org/10.1530/ERC-17-0004.
43. Mete Ö, Cintosun A, Pressman IS, Sylvia L. Epidemiology and biomarker profile of pituitary adenohypophysial tumors. Modern Pathology. Published online 2018. https://doi.org/10.1038/S41379-018-0016-8.
44. Chemaitilly W, Armstrong GT, Gajjar A, Hudson MM. Hypothalamic-pituitary axis dysfunction in survivors of childhood CNS tumors: importance of systematic follow-up and early endocrine consultation. J Clin Oncol. Published online 2016. https://doi.org/10.1200/JCO.2016.70.1847.
45. Sylvia L, Mete Ö. Hypothalamic endocrine tumors: an update. J Clin Med. Published online 2019. https://doi.org/10.3390/JCM8101741.
46. Zada G, Lin N, Ojerholm E, Ramkissoon S, Laws ER. Craniopharyngioma and other cystic epithelial lesions of the sellar region: a review of clinical, imaging, and histopathological relationships. Neurosurg Focus. Published online 2010. https://doi.org/10.3171/2010.2.FOCUS09318.
47. Müller HL. Craniopharyngioma. Endocr Rev. Published online 2014. https://doi.org/10.1210/ER.2013-1115.
48. Iersel L van, Brokke KE, Adan RAH, Bulthuis L, Akker ELT van den, Santen HM van. Pathophysiology and individualized treatment of hypothalamic obesity following craniopharyngioma and other suprasellar tumors: a systematic review. Endocr Rev. Published online 2018. https://doi.org/10.1210/ER.2018-00017.
49. Zacharia BE, Bruce SS, Goldstein HE, Malone H, Neugut AI, Bruce JN. Incidence, treatment and survival of patients with craniopharyngioma in the surveillance, epidemiology and end results program. Neuro Oncol. Published online 2012. https://doi.org/10.1093/NEUONC/NOS142.

50. Karavitaki N, Brufani C, Warner J, et al. Craniopharyngiomas in children and adults: systematic analysis of 121 cases with long-term follow-up. Clin Endocrinol (Oxf). Published online 2005. https://doi.org/10.1111/J.1365-2265.2005.02231.X.
51. Duff J, Meyer FB, Ilstrup DM, Laws ER, Schleck CD, Scheithauer BW. Long-term outcomes for surgically resected craniopharyngiomas. Neurosurgery. Published online 2000. https://doi.org/10.1097/00006123-200002000-00007.
52. Müller HL, Merchant TE, Warmuth-Metz M, Martínez-Barberá JP, Puget S. Craniopharyngioma. Nat Rev Dis Primers. Published online 2019. https://doi.org/10.1038/S41572-019-0125-9.
53. Mortini P, Losa M, Pozzobon G, et al. Neurosurgical treatment of craniopharyngioma in adults and children: early and long-term results in a large case series. J Neurosurg. Published online 2011. https://doi.org/10.3171/2010.11.JNS10670.
54. Cavicchiolo ME, Opocher E, Daverio M, et al. Diencephalic syndrome as sign of tumor progression in a child with neurofibromatosis type 1 and optic pathway glioma: a case report. Childs Nervous System. Published online 2013. https://doi.org/10.1007/S00381-013-2109-5.
55. Marec-Bérard P, Szathmári A, Faure-Conter C, Mottolèse C, Berlier P, Frappaz D. Improvement of diencephalic syndrome after partial surgery of optic chiasm glioma. Pediatr Blood Cancer. Published online 2009. https://doi.org/10.1002/PBC.22085.
56. Sawamura Y, Kamada K, Kamoshima Y, et al. Role of surgery for optic pathway/hypothalamic astrocytomas in children. Neuro Oncol. Published online 2008. https://doi.org/10.1215/15228517-2008-033.
57. Yumuşakhuylu AC, Binnetoğlu A, Topuz MF, Bozkurtlar E, Bağlam T, Sarı M. Syndrome of inappropriate antidiuretic hormone secretion associated with olfactory neuroblastoma. J Craniofac Surg. Published online 2013. https://doi.org/10.1097/SCS.0B013E3182A41C52.
58. Parvizi J, Le S, Foster BL, et al. Gelastic epilepsy and hypothalamic hamartomas: neuroanatomical analysis of brain lesions in 100 patients. Brain. Published online 2011. https://doi.org/10.1093/BRAIN/AWR235.
59. Chan YM, Fenoglio-Simeone KA, Paraschos S, et al. Central precocious puberty due to hypothalamic hamartomas correlates with anatomic features but not with expression of GnRH, TGFα, or KISS1. Horm Res Paediatr. Published online 2010. https://doi.org/10.1159/000308162.
60. Alomari S, Houshiemy MN el, Bsat S, Moussalem C, Allouh MZ, Omeis I. Hypothalamic hamartomas: a comprehensive review of the literature—Part 1: Neurobiological features, clinical presentations and advancements in diagnostic tools. Clinical neurology and neurosurgery (Dutch-Flemish ed Print). Published online 2020. https://doi.org/10.1016/J.CLINEURO.2020.106076.
61. Castaño CC, Mota D la, Valle MG del, et al. [Hypothalamic hamartoma in paediatric patients: clinical characteristics, outcomes and review of the literature]. Neurología. Published online 2012. https://doi.org/10.1016/J.NRL.2011.12.008.
62. Ntali G, Capatina CAM. Updating the landscape for functioning gonadotroph tumors. Medicina (B Aires). Published online 2022. https://doi.org/10.3390/MEDICINA58081071.
63. Castelo-Branco C, Pino M del, Valladares E. Ovarian hyperstimulation, hyperprolactinaemia and LH gonadotroph adenoma. Reprod Biomed Online. Published online 2009. https://doi.org/10.1016/S1472-6483(10)60065-X.
64. Coté DJ, Smith TR, Sandler CN, et al. Functional gonadotroph adenomas: case series and report of literature. Neurosurgery. Published online 2016. https://doi.org/10.1227/NEU.0000000000001188.
65. Ilie MD, Raverot G. Treatment options for gonadotroph tumors: current state and perspectives. J Clin Endocrinol Metab. Published online 2020. https://doi.org/10.1210/CLINEM/DGAA497.
66. He Y, Gao YT, Sun L. Functioning gonadotroph adenoma with hyperestrogenemia and ovarian hyperstimulation in a reproductive-aged woman: A case report and review of literature. World J Clin Cases. Published online 2023. https://doi.org/10.12998/WJCC.V11.I6.1341.

67. Papanikolaou N, Millar O, Coulden A, et al. Clinical characteristics of functioning gonadotroph adenoma in women presenting with ovarian hyperstimulation: Audit of UK pituitary centres. Clin Endocrinol (Oxf). Published online 2023. https://doi.org/10.1111/CEN.14949.
68. Ntali G, Căpăţînă C, Grossman A, Karavitaki N. Clinical review: Functioning gonadotroph adenomas. J Clin Endocrinol Metab. Published online 2014. https://doi.org/10.1210/JC.2014-2362.
69. Wang L, Liang H, Deng C, et al. Functioning gonadotroph adenomas in premenopausal women: clinical and molecular characterization and review of the literature. Pituitary. Published online 2022. https://doi.org/10.1007/S11102-021-01205-9.
70. Brauner R, Trivin C, Zerah ML, et al. Diencephalic syndrome due to hypothalamic tumor: a model of the relationship between weight and puberty onset. J Clin Endocrinol Metab. Published online 2006. https://doi.org/10.1210/JC.2006-0322.
71. Clarke MJ, Erickson D, Castro MR, Atkinson JLD. Thyroid-stimulating hormone pituitary adenomas. J Neurosurg. Published online 2008. https://doi.org/10.3171/JNS/2008/109/7/0017.
72. Beck-Peccoz P, Persani L, Mannavola D, Campi I. TSH-secreting adenomas. Best Pract Res Clin Endocrinol Metab. Published online 2009. https://doi.org/10.1016/J.BEEM.2009.05.006.
73. Uvelius E, Höglund P, Valdemarsson S, Siesjö P. An early post-operative ACTH suppression test can safely predict short- and long-term remission after surgery of Cushing's disease. Pituitary. Published online 2018. https://doi.org/10.1007/S11102-018-0902-6.
74. Petersenn S, Beckers A, Ferone D, et al. Therapy of endocrine disease: outcomes in patients with Cushing's disease undergoing transsphenoidal surgery: systematic review assessing criteria used to define remission and recurrence. Eur J Endocrinol. Published online 2015. https://doi.org/10.1530/EJE-14-0883.
75. Flitsch J, Knappe UJ, Lüdecke D. The use of postoperative ACTH levels as a marker for successful transsphenoidal microsurgery in Cushing's disease. Zentralbl Neurochir. Published online 2003. https://doi.org/10.1055/S-2003-37145.
76. Invitti C, Giraldi FP, Martin M de, Cavagnini F. Diagnosis and management of Cushing's syndrome: results of an Italian multicentre study. Study Group of the Italian Society of Endocrinology on the Pathophysiology of the Hypothalamic-Pituitary-Adrenal Axis. J Clin Endocrinol Metab. Published online 1999. https://doi.org/10.1210/JCEM.84.2.5465.
77. Utz AL, Swearingen B, Biller BMK. Pituitary surgery and postoperative management in Cushing's disease. Endocrinol Metab Clin North Am. Published online 2005. https://doi.org/10.1016/J.ECL.2005.01.007.
78. Hameed N, Yedinak CG, Brzana J, et al. Remission rate after transsphenoidal surgery in patients with pathologically confirmed Cushing's disease, the role of cortisol, ACTH assessment and immediate reoperation: a large single center experience. Pituitary. Published online 2013. https://doi.org/10.1007/S11102-012-0455-Z.
79. Nieman LK, Biller BMK, Findling JW, et al. Treatment of Cushing's syndrome: an Endocrine Society Clinical Practice Guideline. J Clin Endocrinol Metab. Published online 2015. https://doi.org/10.1210/JC.2015-1818.
80. Pivonello R, Leo M de, Cozzolino A, Colao A. The treatment of Cushing's disease. Endocr Rev. Published online 2015. https://doi.org/10.1210/ER.2013-1048.
81. Theodoropoulou M, Reincke M. Tumor-directed therapeutic targets in Cushing disease. J Clin Endocrinol Metab. Published online 2018. https://doi.org/10.1210/JC.2018-02080.
82. Renner U, Ciato D, Stalla GK. Recent advances in understanding corticotroph pituitary tumor initiation and progression. F1000Res. Published online 2018. https://doi.org/10.12688/F1000RESEARCH.14789.1.
83. Dahia PLM. The molecular pathogenesis of corticotroph tumors. Endocr Rev. Published online 1999. https://doi.org/10.1210/ER.20.2.136.
84. Dworakowska D, Grossman A. The molecular pathogenesis of corticotroph tumours. Eur J Clin Invest. Published online 2012. https://doi.org/10.1111/J.1365-2362.2011.02621.X.
85. Theodoropoulou M, Arzberger T, Gruebler Y, et al. Expression of epidermal growth factor receptor in neoplastic pituitary cells: evidence for a role in corticotropinoma cells. J Endocrinol. Published online 2004. https://doi.org/10.1677/JOE.1.05616.

86. Sylvia L, Kovacs K, Tindall G, Barrow D, Horváth É, Vecsei P. Cushing's disease associated with an intrasellar gangliocytoma producing corticotrophin-releasing factor. Ann Intern Med. Published online 1984. https://doi.org/10.7326/0003-4819-101-6-789.
87. Marko NF, Hamrahian AH, Weil RJ. Immediate postoperative cortisol levels accurately predict postoperative hypothalamic-pituitary-adrenal axis function after transsphenoidal surgery for pituitary tumors. Pituitary. Published online 2010. https://doi.org/10.1007/S11102-010-0227-6.
88. Wong A, Eloy JA, Couldwell WT, Liu JK. Update on prolactinomas. Part 2: Treatment and management strategies. J Clin Neurosci. Published online 2015. https://doi.org/10.1016/J.JOCN.2015.03.059.
89. Freeman ME, Kanyicska B, Lerant A, Nagy GM. Prolactin: structure, function, and regulation of secretion. Physiol Rev. Published online 2000. https://doi.org/10.1152/PHYSREV.2000.80.4.1523.
90. Soh NAAC, Yaacob NM, Omar J, et al. Global prevalence of macroprolactinemia among patients with hyperprolactinemia: a systematic review and meta-analysis. Int J Environ Res Public Health. Published online 2020. https://doi.org/10.3390/IJERPH17218199.
91. Domingue MÈ, Devuyst F, Alexopoulou O, Corvilain B, Maiter D. Outcome of prolactinoma after pregnancy and lactation: a study on 73 patients. Clin Endocrinol (Oxf). Published online 2014. https://doi.org/10.1111/CEN.12370.
92. Molitch ME. Endocrinology in pregnancy: management of the pregnant patient with a prolactinoma. Eur J Endocrinol. Published online 2015. https://doi.org/10.1530/EJE-14-0848.
93. Maiter D. Management of dopamine agonist-resistant prolactinoma. Neuroendocrinology. Published online 2019. https://doi.org/10.1159/000495775.
94. Chanson P, Maiter D. The epidemiology, diagnosis and treatment of Prolactinomas: the old and the new. Best Pract Res Clin Endocrinol Metab. Published online 2019. https://doi.org/10.1016/J.BEEM.2019.101290.
95. Casanueva FF, Molitch ME, Schlechte J, et al. Guidelines of the Pituitary Society for the diagnosis and management of prolactinomas. Clin Endocrinol (Oxf). Published online 2006. https://doi.org/10.1111/J.1365-2265.2006.02562.X.
96. Мелмед Ш, Casanueva FF, Hoffman AR, et al. Diagnosis and treatment of hyperprolactinemia: an Endocrine Society clinical practice guideline. J Clin Endocrinol Metab. Published online 2011. https://doi.org/10.1210/JC.2010-1692.
97. Auriemma RS, Pirchio R, Pivonello C, Garifalos F, Colao A, Pivonello R. Approach to the patient with prolactinoma. J Clin Endocrinol Metab. Published online 2023. https://doi.org/10.1210/CLINEM/DGAD174.
98. Inder WJ, Jang C, Inder WJ, Jang C. Treatment of prolactinoma. Medicina-lithuania. Published online 2022. https://doi.org/10.3390/MEDICINA58081095.
99. Ciccarelli A, Daly A, Beckers A. The epidemiology of prolactinomas. Pituitary. Published online 2017. https://doi.org/10.1007/S11102-005-5079-0.
100. Fukuhara N, Nishiyama M, Iwasaki Y. Update in pathogenesis, diagnosis, and therapy of prolactinoma. Cancers (Basel). Published online 2022. https://doi.org/10.3390/CANCERS14153604.
101. Giustina A, Barkhoudarian G, Beckers A, et al. Multidisciplinary management of acromegaly: a consensus. Rev Endocr Metab Disord. Published online 2020. https://doi.org/10.1007/S11154-020-09588-Z.
102. Azzalin A, Appin C, Schniederjan M, et al. Comprehensive evaluation of thyrotropinomas: single-center 20-year experience. Pituitary. Published online 2016. https://doi.org/10.1007/S11102-015-0697-7.
103. Beck-Peccoz P, Giavoli C, Lania A. A 2019 update on TSH-secreting pituitary adenomas. J Endocrinol Invest. Published online 2019. https://doi.org/10.1007/S40618-019-01066-X.
104. Tjörnstrand A, Nyström HF. Diagnosis of endocrine disease: diagnostic approach to TSH-producing pituitary adenoma. Eur J Endocrinol. Published online 2017. https://doi.org/10.1530/EJE-16-1029.

105. Losa M, Giovanelli M, Persani L, Mortini P, Faglia G, Beck-Peccoz P. Criteria of cure and follow-up of central hyperthyroidism due to thyrotropin-secreting pituitary adenomas. J Clin Endocrinol Metab. Published online 1996. https://doi.org/10.1210/JCEM.81.8.8768879.
106. Beck-Peccoz P. Thyrotropin-secreting pituitary tumors. Endocrinol Metab Clin North Am. Published online 1996. https://doi.org/10.1210/EDRV-17-6-610.
107. Varsseveld NC van, Bisschop PH, Biermasz NR, Pereira AM, Fliers E, Drent ML. A long-term follow-up study of eighteen patients with thyrotrophin-secreting pituitary adenomas. Clin Endocrinol (Oxf). Published online 2014. https://doi.org/10.1111/CEN.12290.
108. Beck-Peccoz P, Lania A, Beckers A, Chatterjee K, Wémeau JL. 2013 European Thyroid Association guidelines for the diagnosis and treatment of thyrotropin-secreting pituitary tumors. Eur Thyroid J. Published online 2013. https://doi.org/10.1159/000351007.
109. Amlashi FG, Tritos NA. Thyrotropin-secreting pituitary adenomas: epidemiology, diagnosis, and management. Endocrine. Published online 2016. https://doi.org/10.1007/S12020-016-0863-3.
110. Yamada S, Fukuhara N, Horiguchi K, et al. Clinicopathological characteristics and therapeutic outcomes in thyrotropin-secreting pituitary adenomas: a single-center study of 90 cases. J Neurosurg. Published online 2014. https://doi.org/10.3171/2014.7.JNS1471.
111. Turcu AF, Erickson BJ, Lin E, et al. Pituitary stalk lesions: the Mayo Clinic experience. J Clin Endocrinol Metab. Published online 2013. https://doi.org/10.1210/JC.2012-4171.
112. Kurucu N, Akyüz C, Varan A, et al. Primary intracranial germ cell tumors in children 36-year experience of a single center. J Cancer Res Ther. Published online 2020. https://doi.org/10.4103/JCRT.JCRT_314_18.
113. Gao Y, Jiang J, Liu Q. Clinicopathological and immunohistochemical features of primary central nervous system germ cell tumors: a 24-years experience. Int J Clin Exp Pathol. Published online 2014.
114. Fu H, Guo X, Li R, Xing B. Radiotherapy and chemotherapy plus radiation in the treatment of patients with pure intracranial germinoma: a meta-analysis. J Clin Neurosci. Published online 2017. https://doi.org/10.1016/J.JOCN.2017.05.024.
115. Gutenberg A, Bell J, Lupi I, et al. Pituitary and systemic autoimmunity in a case of intrasellar germinoma. Pituitary. Published online 2011. https://doi.org/10.1007/S11102-009-0187-X.
116. Bhimani AD, Barrington NM, Aguilar TM, Arnone GD, Mehta AI. Pituitary germinomas: a multi-institutional study analyzing patient demographics and management patterns. Pituitary. Published online 2020. https://doi.org/10.1007/S11102-020-01042-2.
117. Isono M, Kamida T, Kobayashi H, Shimomura T, Matsuyama J. Clinical features of symptomatic Rathke's cleft cyst. Clin Neurol Neurosurg. Published online 2001. https://doi.org/10.1016/S0303-8467(01)00121-4.
118. Kim JE, Kim JH, Kim OL, et al. Surgical treatment of symptomatic Rathke cleft cysts: clinical features and results with special attention to recurrence. J Neurosurg. Published online 2004. https://doi.org/10.3171/JNS.2004.100.1.0033.
119. Binning MJ, Liu JK, Gannon J, Osborn AG, Couldwell WT. Hemorrhagic and nonhemorrhagic Rathke cleft cysts mimicking pituitary apoplexy. J Neurosurg. Published online 2008. https://doi.org/10.3171/JNS/2008/108/01/0003.
120. Raper D, Besser M. Clinical features, management and recurrence of symptomatic Rathke's cleft cyst. J Clin Neurosci. Published online 2009. https://doi.org/10.1016/J.JOCN.2008.04.023.
121. Komatsu F, Tsugu H, Komatsu M, et al. Clinicopathological characteristics in patients presenting with acute onset of symptoms caused by Rathke's cleft cysts. Acta Neurochir (Wien). Published online 2010. https://doi.org/10.1007/S00701-010-0687-5.
122. Chaiban J, Abdelmannan D, Cohen ML, Selman WR, Arafah BM. Rathke cleft cyst apoplexy: a newly characterized distinct clinical entity. J Neurosurg. Published online 2011. https://doi.org/10.3171/2010.5.JNS091905.
123. Potts MB, Jahangiri A, Lamborn KR, Blevins LS, Kunwar S, Aghi MK. Suprasellar Rathke cleft cysts: clinical presentation and treatment outcomes. Neurosurgery. Published online 2011. https://doi.org/10.1227/NEU.0B013E318228BCEA.

124. Zada G. Rathke cleft cysts: a review of clinical and surgical management. Neurosurg Focus. Published online 2011. https://doi.org/10.3171/2011.5.FOCUS1183.
125. Iannelli A, Martini C, Cosottini M, Castagna M, Bogazzi F, Muscatello L. Rathke's cleft cysts in children: clinical, diagnostic, and surgical features. Childs Nervous System. Published online 2012. https://doi.org/10.1007/S00381-011-1626-3.
126. Trifănescu R, Ansorge O, Wass J, Grossman A, Karavitaki N. Rathke's cleft cysts. Clin Endocrinol (Oxf). Published online 2012. https://doi.org/10.1111/J.1365-2265.2011.04235.X.
127. Zhong W, You C, Jiang S, et al. Symptomatic Rathke cleft cyst. J Clin Neurosci. Published online 2012. https://doi.org/10.1016/J.JOCN.2011.07.022.
128. Han SJ, Rolston JD, Jahangiri A, Aghi MK. Rathke's cleft cysts: review of natural history and surgical outcomes. J Neurooncol. Published online 2014. https://doi.org/10.1007/S11060-013-1272-6.
129. Sala E, Moore JM, Amorin A, et al. Natural history of Rathke's cleft cysts: a retrospective analysis of a two centres experience. Clin Endocrinol (Oxf). Published online 2018. https://doi.org/10.1111/CEN.13744.
130. Kazlauskaite R, Evans AT, Villabona C v, et al. Corticotropin tests for hypothalamic-pituitary- adrenal insufficiency: a metaanalysis. J Clin Endocrinol Metab. Published online 2008. https://doi.org/10.1210/JC.2008-0710.
131. Crowley R, Argese N, Tomlinson J, Stewart PM. Central hypoadrenalism. J Clin Endocrinol Metab. Published online 2014. https://doi.org/10.1210/JC.2014-2476.
132. Ospina NS, Nofal A al, Bancos I, et al. ACTH stimulation tests for the diagnosis of adrenal insufficiency: systematic review and meta-analysis. J Clin Endocrinol Metab. Published online 2016. https://doi.org/10.1210/JC.2015-1700.
133. Fleseriu M, Hashim IA, Karavitaki N, et al. Hormonal replacement in hypopituitarism in adults: an Endocrine Society clinical practice guideline. J Clin Endocrinol Metab. Published online 2016. https://doi.org/10.1210/JC.2016-2118.
134. Guaraldi F, Karamouzis I, Berardelli R, et al. Secondary adrenal insufficiency: where is it hidden and what does it look like? Front Horm Res. Published online 2016. https://doi.org/10.1159/000443915.
135. Bornstein SR, Allolio B, Arlt W, et al. Diagnosis and treatment of primary adrenal insufficiency: an Endocrine Society clinical practice guideline. J Clin Endocrinol Metab. Published online 2016. https://doi.org/10.1210/JC.2015-1710.
136. Paragliola RM, Corsello SM. Secondary adrenal insufficiency: from the physiopathology to the possible role of modified-release hydrocortisone treatment. Minerva Endocrinol. Published online 2018. https://doi.org/10.23736/S0391-1977.17.02701-8.
137. Gruber L, Bancos I. Secondary adrenal insufficiency: recent updates and new directions for diagnosis and management. Endocrine Practice. Published online 2021. https://doi.org/10.1016/J.EPRAC.2021.09.011.
138. Kumar R, Wassif W, Pathol C. Adrenal insufficiency. J Clin Pathol. Published online 2022. https://doi.org/10.1136/JCLINPATH-2021-207895.
139. Bereket A. Postoperative and long-term complications of craniopharyngioma. Horm Res Pediatr. 2020;93:497–509.
140. Manuylova E, Calvi L, Vates G, Hastings C, Shafig I. Monitoring serum cortisol level after transsphenoidal surgery for pituitary adenoma predicts hypothalamic-pituitary-adrenal function despite intraoperative dexamethasone use. Endocr Pract. 2015;21(8):897–902.
141. Prete A, Corsello SM, Salvatori R. Current best practice in the management of patients after pituitary surgery. Ther Adv Endocrin Metab. 2017;8(3):33–48.
142. Taplin C, Cowel C, Silink M, Ambler G. Fludcortisone therapy in cerebral salt wasting. Pediatrics. 2006;118(6):1904–8.
143. Jones DP. Syndrome of inappropriate secretion of antidiuretic hormone and hyponatremia. Pediatr Rev. 2018;39(1):27–35.

144. Rabich S, Flynn M, Pelley E. Daily sodium monitoring and fluid intake protocol: preventing recurrent hospitalization in adipsic diabetes insipidus. Journal of Endocrine Society. 2019;3(5):882–6.
145. Perkes I, Menon D, Nott M, Baguley I. Paroxysmal sympathetic hyperactivity after acquired brain injury: a review of diagnostic criteria. Brain Inj. Published online 2011. https://doi.org/10.3109/02699052.2011.589797.
146. Fernández-Ortega JF, Prieto-Palomino MÁ, García-Caballero M, López JLG, Quesada-García G, Baguley I. Paroxysmal sympathetic hyperactivity after traumatic brain injury: clinical and prognostic implications. J Neurotrauma. Published online 2012. https://doi.org/10.1089/NEU.2011.2033.
147. Choi HA, Jeon S, Samuel S, Allison TA, Lee K. Paroxysmal sympathetic hyperactivity after acute brain injury. Curr Neurol Neurosci Rep. Published online 2013. https://doi.org/10.1007/S11910-013-0370-3.
148. Lump D, Moyer M. Paroxysmal sympathetic hyperactivity after severe brain injury. Curr Neurol Neurosci Rep. Published online 2014. https://doi.org/10.1007/S11910-014-0494-0.
149. Samuel S, Allison TA, Lee K, Choi HA. Pharmacologic management of paroxysmal sympathetic hyperactivity after brain injury. J Neurosci Nurs. Published online 2016. https://doi.org/10.1097/JNN.0000000000000207.
150. Meyfroidt G, Baguley I, Menon D. Paroxysmal sympathetic hyperactivity: the storm after acute brain injury. Lancet Neurology. Published online 2017. https://doi.org/10.1016/S1474-4422(17)30259-4.
151. Jafari AA, Shah M, Mirmoeeni S, et al. Paroxysmal sympathetic hyperactivity during traumatic brain injury. Clinical neurology and neurosurgery (Dutch-Flemish ed Print). Published online 2022. https://doi.org/10.1016/J.CLINEURO.2021.107081.
152. Yuan P, Zhu H, Chen H, et al. Dexmedetomidine attenuates acute paroxysmal sympathetic hyperactivity. Oncotarget. Published online 2017. https://doi.org/10.18632/ONCOTARGET.16920.
153. Branstetter JW, Ohman K, Johnson DW, Gilbert BW. Management of paroxysmal sympathetic hyperactivity with dexmedetomidine and propranolol following traumatic brain injury in a pediatric patient. J Pediatr Intensive Care. Published online 2020. https://doi.org/10.1055/S-0039-1698758.
154. Shald EA, Reeder JA, Finnick M, et al. Pharmacological treatment for paroxysmal sympathetic hyperactivity. Crit Care Nurse. Published online 2020. https://doi.org/10.4037/CCN2020348.
155. Tu J, Reeve J, Deane AM, Plummer MP. Pharmacological management of Paroxysmal Sympathetic Hyperactivity (PSH): a scoping review. J Neurotrauma. Published online 2021. https://doi.org/10.1089/NEU.2020.7597.
156. Carozza RB, Mohanty D, Wolf M, Martin E, Anderson J, Pagano LM. Paroxysmal sympathetic hyperactivity: development of a pediatric clinical practice guideline. Hosp Pediatr. Published online 2023. https://doi.org/10.1542/HPEDS.2023-007261.
157. Jerousek CR, Reinert JP. The role of dexmedetomidine in paroxysmal sympathetic hyperactivity: a systematic review. Ann Pharmacother. Published online 2023. https://doi.org/10.1177/10600280231194708.

GPSR Compliance

*The European Union's (EU) General Product Safety Regulation (GPSR) is a set of rules that requires consumer products to be safe and our obligations to ensure this.*

*If you have any concerns about our products, you can contact us on ProductSafety@springernature.com*

In case Publisher is established outside the EU, the EU authorized representative is:

Springer Nature Customer Service Center GmbH
Europaplatz 3
69115 Heidelberg, Germany

**Batch number: 10732090**

Printed by Printforce, the Netherlands